T0226472

Quality Control in the Age of Risk Management

Editors

JAMES O. WESTGARD
STEN WESTGARD

CLINICS IN LABORATORY MEDICINE

www.labmed.theclinics.com

March 2013 • Volume 33 • Number 1

ELSEVIER

1600 John F. Kennedy Boulevard • Suite 1800 • Philadelphia, Pennsylvania, 19103-2899

http://www.theclinics.com

CLINICS IN LABORATORY MEDICINE Volume 33, Number 1
March 2013 ISSN 0272-2712, ISBN-13: 978-1-4557-7110-3

Editor: Teia Stone

Reprints. For copies of 100 or more, of articles in this publication, please contact the Commercial Reprints Department, Elsevier Inc., 360 Park Avenue South, New York, New York 10010-1710. Tel. (212) 633-3813, Fax: (212) 462-1935, E-mail: reprints@elsevier.com.

Clinics in Laboratory Medicine (ISSN 0272-2712) is published quarterly by Elsevier Inc., 360 Park Avenue South, New York, NY 10010-1710. Months of issue are March, June, September, and December. Business and Editorial offices: 1600 John F. Kennedy Blvd., Suite 1800, Philadelphia, PA 19103-2899. Periodicals postage paid at NewYork, NY and additional mailing offices. Subscription prices are $240.00 per year (US individuals), $382.00 per year(US institutions), $129.00(US students), $291.00 per year (Canadian individuals), $483.00 per year (foreign institutions), $177.00 (foreign students). Foreign air speed delivery is included in all Clinics subscription prices. All prices are subject to change without notice. POSTMASTER: Send address changes to *Clinics in Laboratory Medicine*, Elsevier Health Sciences Division, Subscription Customer Service, 3251 Riverport Lane, Maryland Heights, MO 63043. **Customer Service: 1-800-654-2452 (US). From outside of the US and Canada, call 1-314-447-8871. Fax: 1-314-447-8029. E-mail: journalscustomer service-usa@elsevier.com (for print support) or journalsonlinesupport-usa@elsevier.com (for online support).**

Clinics in Laboratory Medicine is covered in *EMBASE/Exerpta Medica, MEDLINE/PubMed (Index Medicus), Cinahl, Current Contents/Clinical Medicine, BIOSIS* and *ISI/BIOMED.*

Printed and bound by CPI Group (UK) Ltd, Croydon, CR0 4YY

Transferred to digital print 2013

Contributors

EDITORS

JAMES O. WESTGARD, PhD, FACB
Emeritus Professor, Department of Pathology and Laboratory Medicine, University of Wisconsin; President, Westgard QC, Inc, Madison, Wisconsin

STEN WESTGARD, MS
Director, Client Services and Technology, Westgard QC, Madison, Wisconsin

AUTHORS

DAVID ARMBRUSTER, PhD, DABCC, FACB
Global Scientific Affairs, Abbott Diagnostics, Abbott Park, Illinois

R. NEILL CAREY, PhD, FACB
Consultant, Salisbury, Maryland

DANIEL A. DALENBERG, BS
Technical Specialist II, Department of Laboratory Medicine and Pathology, Mayo Clinic, Rochester, Minnesota

TERESA P. DARCY, MD, MMM
Associate Professor of Pathology and Laboratory Medicine, Department of Pathology and Laboratory Medicine, University of Wisconsin School of Medicine and Public Health, Madison, Wisconsin

PAUL D'ORAZIO, PhD
Research and Development, Instrumentation Laboratory, Bedford, Massachusetts

SHARON S. EHRMEYER, PhD, MT(ASCP)
Professor, Department of Pathology and Laboratory Medicine, University of Wisconsin School of Medicine and Public Health, Madison, Wisconsin

JAY B. JONES, PhD, DABCC
Director of Chemistry and Regional Laboratories, Division of Laboratory Medicine 01-31, Geisinger Medical Center, Geisinger Health System, Danville, Pennsylvania

GEORGE G. KLEE, MD, PhD
Professor of Laboratory Medicine and Pathology, College of Medicine, Mayo Clinic, Rochester, Minnesota

SOHRAB MANSOURI, PhD
Research and Development, Instrumentation Laboratory, Bedford, Massachusetts

CURTIS A. PARVIN, PhD
Manager of Advanced Statistical Research, Quality Systems Division, Bio-Rad Laboratories, Plano, Texas

NILS B. PERSON, PhD, FACB
Clinical Chemist, Madison, New Jersey

PATRICIA G. SCHRYVER, BS
IT Technical Specialist I, Department of Health Sciences Research, Mayo Clinic, Rochester, Minnesota

JOELY A. STRASESKI, PhD, DABCC
Assistant Professor, University of Utah and ARUP Laboratories, Salt Lake City, Utah

FREDERICK G. STRATHMANN, PhD, DABCC (CC, TC)
Assistant Professor, University of Utah and ARUP Laboratories, Salt Lake City, Utah

STACY E. WALZ, PhD, MT(ASCP)
Assistant Professor of Clinical Laboratory Science, Department of Clinical Laboratory Sciences, Arkansas State University, State University, Arkansas

JAMES O. WESTGARD, PhD, FACB
Emeritus Professor, Department of Pathology and Laboratory Medicine, University of Wisconsin; President, Westgard QC, Inc, Madison, Wisconsin

STEN WESTGARD, MS
Director, Client Services and Technology, Westgard QC, Madison, Wisconsin

JOHN YUNDT-PACHECO, MSCS
Scientific Fellow, Quality Systems Division, Bio-Rad Laboratories, Plano, Texas

Contents

> Six Sigma provides data-driven techniques that can enhance and improve the EP23 risk management approach for formulating quality control (QC) Plans. Risk analysis has significant drawbacks in its ability to identify and appropriately prioritize hazards and failure modes for mitigation of risks. Six Sigma quality management is inherently risk oriented on the basis of the required tolerance limits that define defective products. Six Sigma QC tools provide a quantitative assessment of method performance and an objective selection/design of statistical QC procedures. Furthermore, the observed sigma performance of a method is useful for prioritizing the need for development of QC plans.

> This article proposes analytic performance goals for five quality indicators: precision, trueness, linearity, detection limits, and consistency across instruments and time. We defined our goals using methods linked to clinical practice data. Goals for desirable precision and trueness are based on biological variation. Linearity goals are related to total error recommendations. Detection limit goals are derived from 0.1 percentile of patient values. Goals for consistency are derived from the variability of distributions of patient test values. Data were collected and evaluated for each of these quality indicators for 46 chemistry tests measured on the Roche cobas 8000 analyzer.

> A methodology for computing the maximum expected number of unreliable patient results produced because of an out-of-control condition for a given quality control strategy is presented along with strategies for changing the expected number of unreliable results produced and reported. The expected number of unreliable patient results reported before and after the last accepted quality control evaluation before the detection of an out-of-control condition are discussed and used as design criteria for quality control strategies that meet a laboratory's risk criteria.

> In this article, the process used to develop and validate an integrated quality-control system for a cartridge-based, point-of-care system for critical care analysis is outlined. Application of risk management principles has resulted in a quality control system using a combination of statistical quality control with onboard reference solutions and failure pattern recognition used to flag common failure modes during the analytical phase of the testing process. A combination of traditional external quality control,

integrated quality control to monitor ongoing instrument functionality, operator training, and other laboratory-implemented monitors is most effective in controlling known failure modes during the testing process.

Statistical Quality Control Procedures

James O. Westgard

The right quality control (QC) should ensure the detection of important errors. Statistical QC (SQC) should be included in all QC plans. The Clinical and Laboratory Standards Institute (CLSI) C24A3 provides guidance for the application of SQC in medical laboratories. It describes a QC planning process and provides an SQC selection tool that relates the sigma-metric of a testing process to the medically important systematic error and the rejection characteristics of different SQC procedures. Once the right SQC has been selected, the laboratory must implement SQC right. CLSI C24A3 also provides guidance for establishing run length and control limits.

David Armbruster

Testing quality control samples is routine in the clinical laboratory but typically these are precision controls that monitor only the reproducibility (random error) of an assay and not trueness/bias (systematic error). To assess bias, accuracy controls that address both systematic error (trueness) and random error (precision) are needed. A properly prepared trueness control can be used to assess both bias and precision, as accuracy is defined by both random and systematic error. Providers of reference materials, such as metrology institutes and manufacturers are best suited to provide accuracy controls.

R. Neill Carey

Quality control (QC) procedures incorporating patient means, or average of normals (AoN) algorithms, have been used in hematology laboratories and large reference laboratories for decades to monitor analytical processes during the periods between the testing of reference sample QC materials. With the advent of middleware that includes AoN capability, these QC procedures are now available to many more laboratories, including medium-sized hospital laboratories. AoN procedures can improve the control of tests that have low "sigma-metrics," such as electrolytes, where relatively low numbers of patient results can be averaged to provide a high probability of detecting medically significant errors. QC of nearly one-third of the tests whose AoN capabilities have been studied would possibly benefit from AoN procedures in medium-sized laboratories. To obtain satisfactory performance, laboratories must tailor the applications of AoN procedures to their particular volumes and test characteristics.

Joely A. Straseski and Frederick G. Strathmann

As the clinical laboratory attempts to manage and mitigate risk, individual patient results can be a useful complement to routine quality-control materials. Patient results can be used to detect error or identify potential testing complications at all phases of the total testing process. Patient-specific data algorithms include delta checks, tests to verify specimen or tube type, absurdity checks, and result-based reporting. Delta checks are highlighted because they can uniquely point to issues all along the testing cycle, from preanalytical to postanalytical concerns. When used properly, patient results can work to minimize risk and increase the quality of individual patient results.

Autoverification is rapidly expanding with increased functionality provided by middleware tools. It is imperative that autoverification of laboratory test results be viewed as a process evolving into a broader, more sophisticated form of decision support, which will require strategic planning to form a foundational tool set for the laboratory. One must strategically plan to expand autoverification in the future to include a vision of instrument-generated order interfaces, reflexive testing, and interoperability with other information systems. It is hoped that the observations, examples, and opinions expressed in this article will stimulate such short-term and long-term strategic planning.

Post-analytical laboratory processes have been considered to be less prone to error than preanalytical processes because of the widespread adoption of laboratory automation and interfaced laboratory reporting. Quality monitors and controls for the post-analytical process have focused on critical result notification, meeting established turnaround time goals, and review of changed reports. The rapid increase in the adoption of electronic health records has created a new role for laboratory professionals in the management of patient test results. Laboratory professionals must interface with the clinical side of the health care team in establishing quality control for post-analytical processes, particularly in high-risk transitions of care.

CLINICS IN LABORATORY MEDICINE

Preface

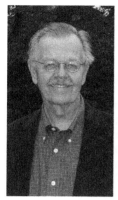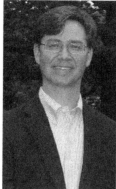

James O. Westgard, PhD, FACB *and* Sten Westgard, MS
Editors

This issue of *Clinics in Laboratory Medicine*, with a focus on "Quality Control (QC) Clinic," addresses changes that are occurring in QC in medical laboratories. In 2012, a new option for satisfying the Clinical Laboratory Improvement Amendments (CLIA) requirements for QC was endorsed by Centers for Medicare and Medicaid Services (CMS). This option follows a new Clinical and Laboratory Standards Institute (CLSI) guideline EP23A, "Laboratory Quality Control Based on Risk Management," that was published in late 2011. CLSI EP23A describes a methodology to identify failure modes, assess their risks, and develop a QC plan that is assembled from a wide variety of control mechanisms in a recommended "QC toolbox." This new approach represents a major change and laboratories will need to invest time and effort to understand the pros and cons of both the new risk management tools and the "old" traditional QC tools.

The first article provides some perspective on quality management and risk management and how they should fit together in a system for Analytical Quality Management. The second article provides an introduction to the CLSI EP23A approach. The author, Nils Person, is a member of the committee that developed EP23A, and he provides an "inside" perspective on both the CLSI guidance and the industry's interests in improving QC. Nils has worked both in clinical laboratories and in industry and has a long-term interest in QC applications. In the next article, Sharon Ehrmeyer provides the background on the regulatory environment and the changes in QC practices that have led to the current situation. The next article describes how Six Sigma principles and concepts can be related to risk management and how Sigma-metrics can help laboratories prioritize applications to develop QC Plans.

In industry, the priority for mitigating risks is to first "design for safety" to reduce and hopefully eliminate the occurrence of failures and medically important errors. In the laboratory, that priority translates to the validation of safety characteristics. Next, Daniel Dalenberg, Patricia Schryver, and George Klee address the importance of

Clin Lab Med 33 (2013) xi–xii
http://dx.doi.org/10.1016/j.cll.2012.11.010
0272-2712/13/$ – see front matter © 2013 Published by Elsevier Inc.   **labmed.theclinics.com**

"safety characteristics" (ie, precision, bias, reportable range, detection limit, comparability of test results) that are critical for assuring that analytical performance is acceptable for the intended use of a laboratory test. A second mitigation strategy is to detect failures to apply corrective actions. That, of course, is the purpose of a laboratory QC Plan. In another article in this issue, John Yundt-Pacheco and Curtis Parvin describe how the performance of control mechanisms can be evaluated to assure that medically important errors will be detected.

Sorab Mansouri and Paul D'Orazio bring a manufacturer's perspective and experience to their discussion of built-in controls. Laboratory users need to understand how manufacturers develop and validate the controls that are built into our analytic systems today. Following that article is a more detailed discussion of Statistical QC, particularly the guidance from the CLSI C24A3 document and some illustrations on the selection of SQC procedures on the basis of Sigma-metrics. David Armbruster discusses trueness controls and the issues of traceability and reference materials. David provides insights from industry as well as from participation in many national and international expert groups.

Patient population controls are described in the article by Neill Carey. Carey has been involved with several CLSI committees and has chaired the committee for EP15. Individual patient controls are addressed by Joely Straseski and Frederick Strathmann. Their work with delta checks is particularly relevant because that is one of the highly recommended controls in the EP23A toolbox.

Jay Jones addresses the issues of implementing controls and the need for informatics support to provide efficient operation for autoverification. Jay works with a large health care network with integrated laboratory services and provides a vision for a comprehensive quality control system. Finally, patient safety and post-analytical errors are addressed by Stacy Walz and Teresa Darcy. Along with traditional issues of critical result reporting and turnaround times, the adoption of the electronic health record creates new issues, particularly in high-risk transitions of care, such as the discharge of patients when laboratory results are pending.

We thank the authors for their timely contributions and helpful advice on changing QC practices in this new era of risk management.

James O. Westgard, PhD, FACB
Department of Pathology and Laboratory Medicine
University of Wisconsin
Madison, WI 53705, USA
Westgard QC, Inc
Madison, WI 53717, USA

Sten Westgard, MS
Director, Client Services and Technology
Westgard QC
7614 Gray Fox Trail
Madison, WI 53717, USA

E-mail addresses:
james@westgard.com (J.O. Westgard)
sten@westgard.com (S. Westgard)

Perspectives on Quality Control, Risk Management, and Analytical Quality Management

James O. Westgard, PhD[a,b],*

KEYWORDS

- Risk management • Statistical quality control • Quality control plan • CLSI EP23A
- CLSI C24A3 • ISO 14971

KEY POINTS

- New risk management practices for developing QC Plans should be integrated with existing error management practices to provide an efficient and effective system for analytical quality management.
- The heart of risk management is risk assessment, which depends on identifying potential causes of errors and estimating their risk by their probability of occurrence, the severity of harm, and the detection capability of QC, then evaluating the acceptability of risks.
- Industrial risk management generally uses a 3-factor model that includes occurrence, severity, and detection, whereas Clinical and Laboratory Standards Institute EP23A (Evaluation Protocol 23A) guideline recommends a 2-factor model that includes the probability of occurrence of harm and the severity of harm.
- In a medical laboratory, occurrence should be controlled first by the validation of safety characteristics (eg, precision, bias, reportable range, detection limit).
- Detection should be optimized by designing statistical QC procedures according to the quality required for the intended use of the test and the precision and bias observed for a measurement procedure. Harm should be reduced by detection of medically important errors followed by corrective actions and disclosure of information for safety.
- Statistical QC is still a critical part of any QC Plan to assure effective detection of medically important errors.

BACKGROUND

In October, 2011, the Clinical and Laboratory Standards Institute (CLSI) published the long-awaited EP23A (Evaluation Protocol 23A) guideline on laboratory quality control (QC) based on risk management.[1] On November 4, 2011, the Centers for Medicare

---

[a] Department of Pathology and Laboratory Medicine, University of Wisconsin, Madison, WI 53705, USA; [b] Westgard QC, Inc., 7614 Gray Fox Trail, Madison, WI 53717, USA
* Department of Pathology and Laboratory Medicine, University of Wisconsin, Madison, WI 53705.
E-mail address: james@westgard.com

Clin Lab Med 33 (2013) 1–14
http://dx.doi.org/10.1016/j.cll.2012.10.003   labmed.theclinics.com

and Medicaid Services (CMS) issued a formal announcement of adoption of EP23A as a voluntary QC option under the Clinical Laboratory Improvement Amendments (CLIA) QC policy.[2] CMS specified that the default QC requirement of 2 levels of external QC per day of patient testing would remain if EP23A is not used and that equivalent QC (EQC) would be eventually phased out. On March 9, 2012, CMS confirmed that new CLIA policy would be called the individualized QC plan (IQCP),[3] stating:

> The guidance and concepts of IQCP are a formal representation and compilation of many things laboratories currently do for quality which are already included in CLIA. It is the 'Right QC!' IQCP permits the laboratory to customize its QC plan according to environment, reagents, testing personnel, specimens, and test system, as long as the [I]QCP provides equivalent quality testing.

Welcome to the world of risk management and the right QC.

WHAT IS THE RIGHT QC?

There is no definition of the right QC in the CLSI EP23A document, but in advertising EP23A, CLSI has described right QC as follows:

> 'The Right QC' in today's hospital laboratory is the quality control plan that's right for you! It's made up of many controls that are customized to your individual needs. Controls based on your institution. Controls that capitalize on a variety of measures aimed at preventing errors, detecting weaknesses, and minimizing risk.

I argue that the right QC is what is right for your patients, not what is right for you. The QC plan needs to be customized to meet the needs of your patients, which may be more demanding than the minimum requirements for compliance with the CLIA regulations.

A better definition of the right QC can be found in the CLIA 493.1256 standard on control procedures[4]:

> (a) Laboratory is responsible for having control procedures that monitor the accuracy and precision of the complete analytical process.
> (b) ...must establish the number, type, and frequency of testing control materials...
> (c) The control procedures must[1] detect immediate errors that occur due to test system failure, adverse environmental conditions, and operation performance[2]; Monitor over time the accuracy and precision of test performance that may be influenced by changes in test system performance and environmental conditions, and variance in operator performance.

Add to this definition the guidance from ISO 15189, the global standard from the International Organization for Standardization (ISO) for medical laboratories[5]:

> 5.6.1 The laboratory shall design internal quality control procedures that verify the attainment of the intended quality of results.

In ISO terminology, "intended quality" is related to the quality goal or quality requirement for the test, which in turn depends on the precision and accuracy of the method.

> 5.5 The performance specifications for each procedure used in an examination shall relate to the intended use of that procedure.

Together, ISO and CLIA provide guidance for the selection or design of the right QC according to the intended quality of test results, the precision and bias of the measurement procedure, and the capability to detect medically important errors.

The right QC is not as simple as "a compilation of the many things laboratories currently do...." The right QC is about what laboratories should do to ensure that patient test results are correct and reliable for their intended use. This goal can be accomplished for statistical QC (SQC) procedures by following the guidance in CLSI C24A3[6] and using the QC planning process and sigma-metric QC selection tool, which are described in that document. For that reason, SQC should be part of every QC plan.

WHAT IS RISK MANAGEMENT?

In principle, risk management is an organized way of assessing what might go wrong and identifying what can be done to mitigate the harm from such failures. Although risk management is new in medical laboratories, it has a long history in other industries and is widely used by manufacturers of in vitro diagnostics (IVDs). Some useful references are the texts by Stamatis[7] and McDermott,[8] Krouwer's book on risk management for hospitals,[9] and The Joint Commission's (TJC's) book on proactive risk reduction.[10] Krouwer[11] also published an article on hospital risk management in the pathology literature, and Powers[12] provided a readable discussion of the use of risk management for QC as part of the proceedings from the CLSI conference on the future of QC, which was held in 2005. Garber and Kaufman[13] also describe a common risk management tool, failure modes and effect analysis (FMEA), in their discussion of laboratory quality systems for the twenty-first century.

In practice, risk management involves identifying hazards, or potential sources of harm, determining the failure modes that may lead to harm, prioritizing their importance, then taking actions to mitigate or reduce their impact. The heart of risk management is the estimation of risk from the probability of occurrence of failures, the severity of harm that would result, and the detectability (chance of detecting) of such failures if they occurred.

The 3 factors are commonly called occurrence (OCC), severity (SEV), and detection (DET). Industrial risk models usually include all 3 factors, rank each factor on a scale from 1 to 10, then calculate a risk priority number (RPN) (RPN = OCC*SEV*DET) to describe and prioritize risks. In health care applications, it is common to use a 2-factor model that considers only the probability of occurrence and severity of harm, then rank each factor on scales from 1 to 5 or from 1 to 3, calculate criticality (OCC*SEV) or use a graphical risk acceptability matrix to describe and prioritize risks.

Once risk has been assessed, the next step is to mitigate the effects by preventing or reducing occurrence, improving detection, and reducing harm by corrective actions and disclosure of information for safety. The remaining residual risks must be estimated and their acceptability determined. Ongoing performance is monitored to identify any new failure modes, assess the frequency of occurrence of failures, and identify the need for additional risk mitigations.

WHAT IS THE INDUSTRIAL RISK MANAGEMENT PROCESS?

Fig. 1 provides a general description of the industrial risk management process. There is no one standard process or methodology and risk analysis tools, such as FMEA, are not standardized. For example, a Google search for "risk analysis" yields 521 million results, "risk management" provides 277 million results, "FMEA" gives 4.8 million results, and "FMEA spreadsheet template" 83,000 results. For comparison, "quality control" yields 377 million results, "statistical quality control" gives 14 million, "Westgard Rules" 9720; thus, risk analysis and risk management are as ubiquitous as QC and statistical QC and references to "FMEA spreadsheet templates" are more

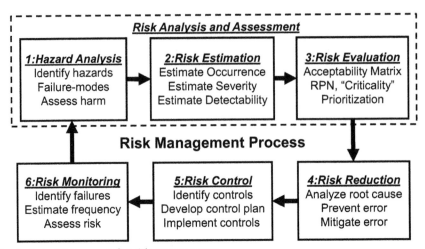

Fig. 1. Industrial process for risk management.

common than references to "Westgard Rules." That is why adoption of risk management techniques for laboratory QC requires much study and deliberation.

Step 1 in the industrial risk management process is hazard analysis and the identification of failure modes that lead to harm. Step 2 (risk estimation) is where occurrence, severity, and detectability are ranked. Step 3 (risk evaluation) compares the estimated risk with some defined acceptable risk, which often involves the use of an acceptability matrix or criticality calculation for 2-factor models (OCC*SEV), or the RPN for 3-factor models. The objective is to identify those high-risk failure modes and prioritize them for mitigation.

Step 4 (risk reduction) starts the risk mitigation activities, which first focus on reducing occurrence by eliminating, preventing, or reducing errors. Step 5 (risk control) focuses on improving detection by identifying controls and developing a control plan. This step is of primary importance in the CLSI EP23A application of risk management for developing QC plans. Step 6 (risk monitoring) is an ongoing effort to identify failures, estimate their frequency, and assess their risk. If new failure modes are identified, then the risk management cycle starts again.

The tool that is commonly used in industrial risk management is called FMEA. This tool is a table that identifies the potential failure modes and their effects, then summarizes the information on occurrence, severity, and detection (including calculations and prioritization of risks), then identifies the risk mitigation strategies. The FMEA table can be large, but is easily constructed and maintained using electronic spreadsheets.

WHAT IS THE ISO 14971 GUIDANCE?

More specific guidance for manufacturers of IVDs is provided in ISO 14971.[14]

Manufacturers of IVDs are required to perform risk analysis as part of the design of any new test or analytical system. ISO 14971[14] is the global standard for guidance to manufacturers on the use of risk management with medical devices. Few medical laboratories have access to that document and must rely on the translation of the ISO guidance via CLSI EP23A document. A general description of the ISO 14971 risk management process is provided in **Fig. 2**. The steps are similar to the generic industrial risk management process, with more emphasis on documenting the manufacturer's risk plan, risk policy, control plan, and risk management report.

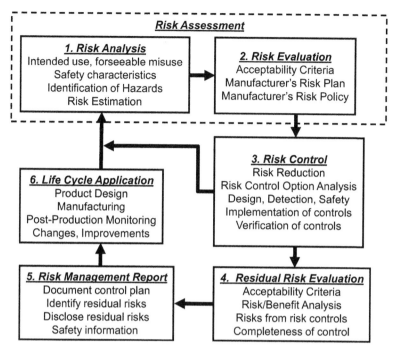

Fig. 2. ISO 14972 risk management process.

There are many terms, such as risk analysis, risk estimation, risk evaluation, and risk assessment, that sound similar but have specific meanings in risk management. For example, risk analysis involves hazard identification and risk estimation. Risk assessment involves risk analysis and risk evaluation. To understand the risk management process, it is necessary to first understand the terminology. **Box 1** provides definitions of many of these terms taken from ISO and CLSI documents.

One important point is that ISO 14971 defines risk as the combination of the probability of occurrence of harm and the severity of harm (ie, a 2-factor model for which an acceptability matrix is recommended for risk evaluation, rather than the use of RPN or criticality). Whereas the common industrial model makes use of probability of occurrence of failures, the ISO model uses the probability of occurrence of harm, which is a more complex term, sufficiently complicated that there is no simple definition in the list of terms. The probability of occurrence of harm begins with the probability of occurrence of a failure, but then also considers whether that failure would be detected, and if not, whether that failure would affect medical decisions and patient care. CLSI EP23A describes the probability of occurrence of harm as the outcome from a sequence of 6 events (ie, the net effect of 6 different probabilities: P1, initiating cause; P2, testing process failure; P3, incorrect result generated; P4, incorrect result reported; P5, misdiagnosis; and P6, hazardous medical action). It seems that the probability of occurrence of failure is represented by P1 and P2 and that P3 and P4 depend on the QC system and its ability to detect the failure and prevent the reporting of erroneous test results. Although use of the probability of occurrence of harm reduces the typical 3-factor model to a 2-factor model, use of that term also makes it more difficult to estimate risk because it encompasses several different probabilities.

Given the complexity of that term, CLSI EP23A recognizes that quantitative estimates are difficult to make and recommends that the probability of occurrence of

---

Box 1
Definitions of terms from ISO and CLSI documents (EP23A and EP18A2)

Criticality: relative measure of the consequences of a failure mode and its frequency of occurrence. Note: combining consequences (severity) with frequency (probability) gives the same measure as defined in risk. (CLSI EP18A2)

Failure: in the broadest sense, a case when the system does not meet the user's expectations. Note 1: failure includes the inability to perform intended functions satisfactorily or within specified performance limits; note 2: errors of measurements and errors of use are subsets of failures. (CLSI EP23A)

Failure mode: manner by which a failure is observed; generally describes the way the failure occurs and its impact on equipment operation. (CLSI EP23A)

FMEA: systematic review of an instrument system or process that examines how failures can affect the instrument or process. Note: FMEA involves identification of potential failure modes, determining the consequences of each failure, and reviewing the control measures implemented to prevent or detect the failure. (CLSI EP18A2)

Harm: physical injury or damage to the health of people, or damage to property or the environment (ISO/TEC Guide 51).

Hazard: potential source of harm (ISO/IEC Guide 51).

Hazard analysis: study of the chains of cause and effect between identified hazards, the hazardous situation to which they might lead, and the resulting harm. Note: the purpose of hazard analysis is to derive sufficient information for the assessment of the risks involved and the identification of preventive measures. (CLSI EP18A2)

Mitigation: an action to lower or eliminate the risk associated with an adverse situation or to prevent the occurrence of future errors. (CLSI EP23A)

QC plan: a document that describes the practices, resources, and sequences of specified activities to control the quality of a particular measuring system or test process to ensure that requirements for its intended purpose are met. (CLSI EP23A)

Residual risk: risk remaining after risk control measures have been taken (ISO 14971).

Risk: combination of probability of occurrence of harm and the severity of that harm (ISO/TEC Guide 51).

Risk analysis: systematic use of available information to identify hazards and to estimate the risk (ISO/TEC Guide 51). Note: risk analysis includes examination of different sequences of events that can produce hazardous situations and harm. (ISO 15189)

Risk assessment: overall process comprising a risk analysis and a risk evaluation (ISO/TEC Guide 51).

Risk estimation: process used to assign values to the probability of occurrence of harm and the severity of harm (ISO 14971)

Risk evaluation: process of comparing the estimated risk against given risk criteria to determine the acceptability of risk (ISO 14971).

Risk management: systematic application of management policies, procedures, and practices to the tasks of analyzing, evaluating, controlling, and monitoring risks (ISO 14971).

Severity: measure of the possible consequences of a hazard (ISO 14971)

---

harm be estimated using a ranking scale of frequent (once per week), probable (once per month), occasional (once per year), remote (once every few years), and improbable (once in the life of the measuring system). Severity is ranked as negligible (inconvenience or temporary discomfort), minor (temporary injury or impairment not requiring professional medical intervention), serious (injury or impairment requiring professional medical intervention), critical (permanent impairment or life-threatening injury), and catastrophic (patient death).

To decide whether risk is acceptable, a risk acceptability matrix is used, as shown in **Fig. 3**. The matrix shows the ranking for severity of harm across the columns and the ranking for probability of occurrence of harm down the rows. The matrix defines certain row-column combinations as acceptable and others as unacceptable, generally separated by a diagonal from the top left to the lower right. The risk acceptability matrices in ISO 14971 and CLSI EP23A are not identical, even although the EP23A document quotes ISO 14971 as its source. That situation is an indicator of the subjectively of risk evaluation, which together with the ranking scales, should alert the laboratory to the qualitative nature of this methodology.

WHAT IS THE METHODOLOGY FOR RISK ANALYSIS IN HEALTH CARE?

There are 2 methodologies that are in use in health care organizations. One has been developed by the Veterans Healthcare Administration and is known as Healthcare FMEA (HFMEA).[15] The other methodology comes from TJC and is called proactive risk reduction.[10] The 2 methodologies use different ranking scales and different prioritization methods, and thus the details of performing risk analysis are different. Of the two, the TJC methodology is more consistent with the CLSI EP23A methodology, whereas the HFMEA is more consistent with the CLSI EP18A2 guidance[16] on risk management techniques to identify and control laboratory error sources. That situation also means that the 2 CLSI documents (EP23A and EP18A2) are not consistent in their guidance on assessing risk. An important lesson here is that as you study available materials on risk management, you encounter inconsistencies that are confusing. It takes time and effort to develop a practical understanding of the risk management process. This situation again suggests that laboratories face a steep learning curve in applying risk management for developing QC plans.

US hospitals are required to perform a formal risk assessment at least once per year to satisfy TJC's requirements for accreditation, and thus many organizations have some background and training in this methodology. The advantages of the TJC methodology are (1) its widespread acceptance in health care organizations, (2) the availability of a detailed manual that describes the process step by step and shows applications of tools and techniques using health care examples, and (3) the use of either 3-factor or 2-factor risk models, depending on what is needed for the intended application.

The TJC proactive risk reduction methodology is described in **Fig. 4**. It is a team problem-solving methodology similar to that used for quality improvement projects

Risk Matrix	Negligible	Minor	Serious	Critical	Catastrophic
Frequent					
Probable		Unacceptable	Risk		
Occasional					
Remote		Acceptable	Risk		
Improbable					

Fig. 3. ISO 14971 risk acceptability matrix showing rankings for severity of harm across columns and rankings for probability of occurrence of harm down rows. Gray cells represent unacceptable risk.

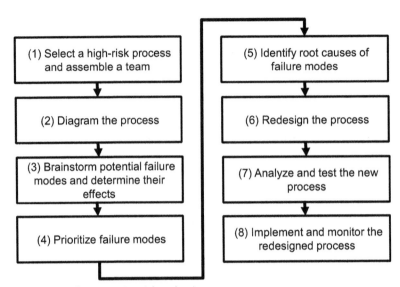

Fig. 4. TJC process for proactive risk reduction.

and uses many of the same tools and techniques. TJC recommends the FMEA tool and provides examples for health care applications. The risk mitigation strategies focus on process redesign with options to (1) eliminate or reduce occurrence, (2) increase detection, and (3) reduce the severity or effects of errors. The redesign option to reduce occurrence is particularly applicable for preanalytical and postanalytical processes, and thus the TJC methodology is more broadly useful than the CLSI EP23A methodology, which focuses primarily on detection (the obvious purpose of a QC plan).

For comparison, the CLSI EP23A methodology is shown in **Fig. 5**. This is not a figure from the EP23A document, but is a summary based on the guidance in the document. EP23A presents several figures to describe the methodology and that information is combined in **Fig. 5** to allow for easier comparison with the TJC methodology. Several of the initial steps parallel the TJC methodology, but there is an important difference in step 3 (risk estimation), for which EP23A recommends a 2-factor risk model that considers only probability of occurrence of harm and severity of harm. Although this strategy is consistent with the ISO 14971 guidance to manufacturers, it is a bad translation of practice for development of QC plans in medical laboratories, given that the primary risk mitigation strategy available in laboratories is to maximize detection (ie, risk control [step 5]). In step 6, EP23A recommends the use of a wide variety of control mechanisms, as shown in the laboratory QC tool box. The selected controls are then assembled together to describe a QC plan (step 7).

WHAT IS A QC PLAN?

According to CLSI EP23A, a QC plan is "a document that describes the practices, resources, and sequences of specified activities to control the quality of a particular measuring system or test process to ensure requirements for its intended purpose are met." There is no standard format and little guidance on what the QC plan should look like, because the idea is new and laboratories have no experience of the process. Conceptually, the QC plan should identify the various controls, specify their frequency, describe corrective actions for recovery, and specify information for disclosure. This

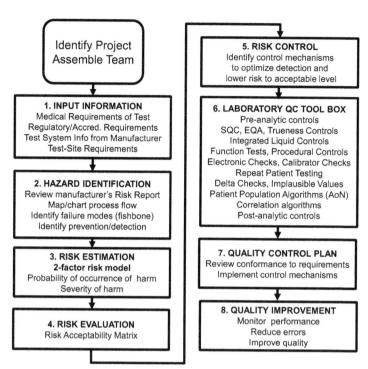

Fig. 5. Summary of the CLSI EP23A methodology for developing a QC plan by risk management.

guidance comes from Krouwer,[9] who chaired the CLSI committee that developed the EP18A2 risk guidance for manufacturers.[16]

Table 1 shows what might be included in a QC plan. Column 1 identifies the controls, organizing them into categories of analyst/operator controls, preanalytical controls, analytical controls, and postanalytical controls. Column 2 specifies frequency or how often the control activities are performed. Column 3 identifies mechanisms for recovery and corrective action. Column 4 identifies information for disclosure or safe use in the terminology of risk management. Columns 3 and 4 are important because harm is mitigated by having good detection followed by corrective actions and disclosure of information for safe use.

The manner in which all this information is written and formatted into a document is left up to the laboratory. As laboratories apply this approach, common formats will likely emerge and at some point there will be recommendations for a standard format for QC plans. Accreditation organizations will drive this standardization of QC plans to simplify and systematize their review during laboratory inspections.

HOW DOES RISK MANAGEMENT FIT TOGETHER WITH ANALYTICAL QUALITY MANAGEMENT?

Risk management, like quality management, can be viewed as a broad and all-encompassing management approach. Like other management approaches, there are fads that come and go, particular approaches that are in vogue for a time, and others that are old and traditional. Risk management is new and on the increase in health care. Some think that risk management QC plans will replace older SQC

Table 1
The information that may be included in a laboratory QC plan

QC Plan	Frequency	Recovery	Disclosure
Analyst/Operator Controls			
Standard operating procedure	Yearly standard operating procedure review	Director review	No
Operator training	Every operator	Supervisor review	No
Operator checklists	Daily	Supervisor review	No
System maintenance	Manufacturer's schedule	Manufacturer repair	No
Operator competency	Yearly	Retrain	No
Preanalytical Controls			
Inspect samples	Every sample	Request new sample	Yes
Analytical Controls			
Electronic checks	Manufacturer	Manufacturer's instructions	No
Function tests	Manufacturer	Manufacturer's instructions	Sample condition
Process tests	Manufacturer	Manufacturer's instructions	No
Calibration checks	Manufacturer/Regulations	Supervisor review	No
SQC	Startup + monitor	Troubleshooting guidelines	No
Trueness control	Calibration	Troubleshooting guidelines	No
Periodic external quality assessment, proficiency testing	Three times per year	Corrective action plan	No
Implausible values	Each test result	Repeat test	Yes
Postanalytical Controls			
Confirm/call critical values	Each critical test	Repeat test	Yes
Monitor turnaround time	Each emergency test	Call test result	Yes

procedures. In reality, risk management adds new tools and techniques that must be integrated with the other tools and techniques that have already been proved to work.

For example, consider a new analytical system. Risk management would consider this system to be a new piece of equipment that should be the subject of a risk assessment project. A project team would be assembled to identify possible failure modes, prioritize their importance, and mitigate high-risk problems. That would be an inefficient and wasteful project because laboratories already have tools, techniques, and protocols that are optimized for this purpose. That is what method validation is all about.

Method validation is an important quality management activity for dealing with the probability of occurrence of failures. Manufacturers design their products to certain specifications, which are then disclosed to the laboratory as part of a manufacturer's information for safety. For analytical systems, information for safety includes performance claims for reportable range, precision, bias, detection limit, analytical specificity, and reference range or cutoff limits. Laboratories have a responsibility to verify that any new method performs as claimed by the manufacturer or to validate that the performance observed satisfies the quality required for the intended use of the tests. The decision to accept or reject a new method or new analytical system is the laboratory's most important strategy for mitigating the occurrence of errors.

Once a new analytical system is implemented for routine service, QC becomes an important strategy. The decision to accept or reject each analytical run becomes critical to ensure quality, or as ISO 15189 says, "to verify the attainment of the intended quality of test results." The laboratory needs to optimize the detection of medically important errors. Here is where the QC plan should fit, but the problem is that the EP23A risk analysis methodology does not require any quantitative assessment of the detection capabilities of the different controls that may be included in a QC plan.

For this reason, SQC should always be included in a QC plan. The detection capabilities of different control rules and different numbers of control measurements are known. That knowledge allows an SQC procedure to be designed according to the quality required for the test and the precision and bias observed for the method, which ensures the detection of medically important systematic errors. SQC is the laboratory's best strategy for optimizing the detection of analytical errors.

Other controls in a QC plan can target specific failure modes, particularly those not covered by SQC. For example, preanalytical problems with lipemic, icteric, or hemolyzed samples require additional controls, such as visual inspection of sample or measurement of sample indices. Postanalytical problems, such as turnaround time and unreported test results at patient discharge, require additional control mechanisms. Manufacturers can provide controls that monitor individual instrument components, functions, and processes. Laboratories can add controls that monitor individual patients, such as delta checks and critical value checks.

The balance between SQC and other controls varies from method to method. That balance can be related to the sigma performance observed for each method. Sigma can be calculated from the quality required for the test (allowable total error [Tea]) and the precision (coefficient of variation [CV]) and accuracy (bias) observed for the method [sigma = (% Tea – % bias)/% CV]. Sigma can then be used to select an appropriate SQC procedure and prioritize the need for other controls. Six-sigma quality management is inherently risk oriented because of its definition of tolerance limits, or quality requirements, and its characterization of quality in terms of the number of defective results.

Current practices for analytical quality management already incorporate strategies to reduce or minimize risk:

- Occurrence is controlled first by validating that precision and accuracy are acceptable for the intended use.
- Detection is optimized by designing the SQC procedure according to the quality required for the test and the precision and bias observed for the method.
- Harm can be reduced by having a good detection system and well-defined recovery and corrective actions, along with disclosure of information for safe use.
- A QC plan should add control mechanisms that complement SQC, particularly controls for preanalytical and postanalytical processes.
- The balance between SQC and other analytical controls in a QC plan can be prioritized by sigma performance.

WHAT IS THE PLAN FOR INTEGRATING RISK ANALYSIS INTO ANALYTICAL QUALITY MANAGEMENT?

After studying the ISO and CLSI documents on risk management and also reading the industrial literature, my perspective is that risk management provides a valuable approach for identifying potential problems and provides a new tool, FMEA, for assessing the risk and importance of these problems. The idea of QC plan expands the laboratory quality system and provides an organized way to incorporate controls for pre-analytical and postanalytical parts of the process. It also provides a model for controlling complex analytical processes on a step-by-step basis (ie, providing a series of individual controls for the critical failure modes throughout the process). New technology and highly complex automated systems require a combination of SQC and specific control mechanisms that are targeted at the weak points in the analytical system.

Given this perspective, a recommendation for integrating risk analysis into our traditional error framework is provided in **Fig. 6**. Step 1 is to define the quality goals or requirements for the intended use of laboratory tests. This step is critical if quality is to become measureable and manageable. Step 2 is to select measurement procedures, or methods, or examination procedures, the precision and accuracy of which satisfies the needs for intended use and the traceability of which leads to comparability

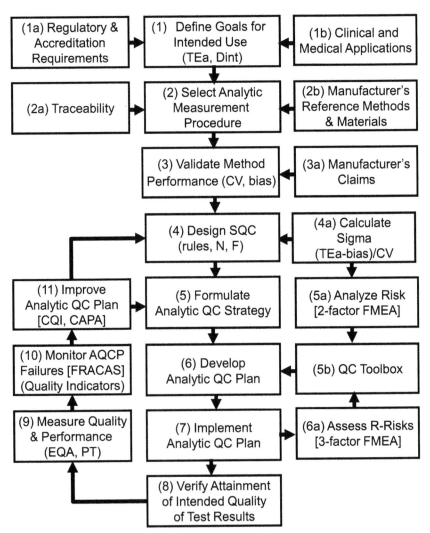

Fig. 6. Integration of risk analysis into a system for analytical quality management.

of test results from method to method. Traceability is a critical characteristic for test results to be useful across laboratories and throughout a geographic area, for treatment guidelines to apply nationally or globally, and for health care to advance beyond the art of medicine to a quality service that is measureable and manageable.

Step 3 is to show with data in the laboratory that the performance observed satisfies the needs for intended use. Method validation is a key part of the laboratory strategy for limiting the occurrence of medically important errors. Given the quality requirement defined in step 1, the precision and accuracy observed in step 3, a sigma-metric can be calculated and used to characterize analytical quality on the sigma scale and guide decisions on the acceptability of performance.

The next steps make use of this sigma-metric to optimize QC. Step 4 is the formulation of an overall or total QC strategy to prioritize the need for different controls and also the need for risk analysis. This strategy is particularly important because risk management applications are initially laborious due to the time and effort required both to learn the methodology and to apply it in an objective manner. Step 5 is to design/select SQC procedures. These procedures can be selected using the sigma-metric QC selection tool described in CLSI C24A3.[6]

Step 6 is to identify and assemble the controls into a QC plan. Step 7 is to implement the plan, which requires informatics support to make operation efficient and effective. Step 8 is the operation of the QC plan to verify the attainment of the intended quality of test results.

Steps 9, 10, and 11 involve monitoring quality and measuring performance, identifying failures and areas for improvement, and implementing those improvements. These steps involve making use of internal quality data, as well as external proficiency testing and external quality assessment data. The frequency of errors can be determined for different failure modes, which makes the estimation of risk more quantitative and more reliable. Laboratories need to estimate defect rates to quantify occurrence, then use six-sigma concepts to estimate risk in terms of the number of potentially harmful patient test results that may be produced.[17]

REFERENCES

1. CLSI EP23A. Laboratory quality control based on risk management. Wayne (PA): Clinical and Laboratory Standards Institute; 2011.
2. CMS memorandum: initial plans and policy implementation for Clinical and Laboratory Standards Institute (CLSI) Evaluation Protocol-23 (EP), "laboratory quality control based on risk management," as Clinical Laboratory Improvement Amendment (CLIA) Quality Control (QC) Policy. 2011.
3. CMS memorandum: implementing the Individualized Quality Control Plan (IQCP) for Clinical Laboratory Improvement Amendments (CLIA). 2012.
4. US Centers for Medicare and Medicaid Services (CMS). Medicare, Medicaid, and CLIA programs. Laboratory requirements relating to quality systems and certain personnel qualifications. Final rule. Fed Regist 2003;16:3640–714.
5. ISO 15189. Medical laboratories–particular requirements for quality and competence. Geneva (Switzerland): ISO; 2007.
6. CLSI C24A3. Statistical quality control for quantitative measurement procedures. Wayne (PA): Clinical and Laboratory Standards Institute; 2006.
7. Stamatis DH. Failure mode effect analysis: FMEA from theory to execution. 2nd edition. Milwaukee (WI): ASQ Press; 2003.
8. McDermott RE, Mikulak RJ, Beauregard MR. The basics of FMEA. 2nd edition. New York: CRC Press; 2009.

9. Krouwer JS. Managing risk in hospitals: using integrated fault trees and failure mode effects and criticality analysis. Washington, DC: AACC Press; 2004.

10. The Joint Commission. Failure modes and effects analysis in health care: proactive risk reduction. Oakbrook Terrace (IL): The Joint Commission, Oakbrook Terrace; 2010.

11. Krouwer JS. An improved failure mode effects analysis for hospitals. Arch Pathol Lab Med 2004;128:663–7.

12. Powers DM. Laboratory quality control requirements should be based on risk management principles. Lab Medicine 2005;36:633–8.

13. Garber CC, Kaufman HW. Quality systems for the clinical laboratory in the 21st century. In: Ward-cook KM, Lehmann CA, Shoeff LE, et al, editors. The postanalytical phase. Clinical diagnostic technology: the total testing process, vol. 3. Washington, DC: AACC Press; 2006. p. 1–36.

14. ISO 14971. Medical devices–application of risk management to medical devices. Geneva (Switzerland): ISO; 2007.

15. De Rosier J, Stalhandske E, Bagian JP, et al. Using health care failure mode and effects analysis: the VA national center for patient safety's proactive risk analysis system. Jt Comm J Qual Improv 2002;27:248–67.

16. CLSI EP18A2. Risk management techniques to identify and control laboratory error sources. 2nd edition. Wayne (PA): Clinical and Laboratory Standards Institute; 2009.

17. Westgard JO. Six sigma risk analysis: designing analytic QC plans for the medical laboratory. Madison (WI): Westgard QC; 2011.

Developing Risk-based Quality Control Plans: An Overview of CLSI EP23-A

Nils B. Person, PhD, FACB

KEYWORDS

- Risk management • Statistical quality control • Quality control plan • CLSI EP23-A

KEY POINTS

- Concept of quality control has evolved from primarily monitoring measuring system stability to managing the risk of reporting incorrect patient results.
- Techniques of risk management can be used to develop an individual laboratory quality-control plan. Clinical and Laboratory Standards Institute document EP23-A provides guidance for this process.
- The steps to develop a quality control plan include:
  - Gathering information about the testing process
  - Assessing risk in the process
  - Developing the quality-control plan to mitigate risks
  - Implementing, monitoring, and updating the plan
- A risk-based quality-control plan can cost-effectively manage risk of reporting incorrect results and meet regulatory requirements.

BACKGROUND

For most of the second half of the twentieth century the term quality control (QC) in the clinical laboratory was generally taken to mean the testing of surrogate quality-control samples designed to mimic the characteristics of patient samples and the use of statistical process control techniques to evaluate the results from these samples to detect significant change in the performance of the analytical or measuring system. This concept of QC was incorporated into regulations applied to the clinical laboratory. For example, the Clinical Laboratory Improvement Amendments (CLIA) 1988 regulations in the United States specify a default acceptable QC protocol as:

At least once each day patient specimens are assayed or examined, perform the following for:
i. Each quantitative procedure, include two control materials of different concentrations;

The author is a clinical chemist with 30 years experience involving both the hospital based clinical laboratory and the in vitro diagnostics industry.
Madison, NJ 07940, USA
E-mail address: nils.person@verizon.net

Clin Lab Med 33 (2013) 15–26
http://dx.doi.org/10.1016/j.cll.2012.11.003
0272-2712/13/$ – see front matter © 2013 Elsevier Inc. All rights reserved.

ii. Each qualitative procedure, include a negative and positive control material; or to calibrate the test system.[1]

In the past, the frequency of testing these external QC samples has been, in large part, driven by the stability of the measuring systems. The frequency of testing QC samples was often linked to the concept of the analytical run. QC samples were included in each analytical run to check for changes in the measuring system at the time of the run. When this QC practice was developed, testing in the clinical laboratory was performed on batches of patient samples and the results from the QC samples included in each batch would be checked before release of the patient results. The technology used in the laboratory has since evolved to include increasing levels of automation, the testing process has become continuous rather than a batch process, and the concept of the analytical run has evolved to focus on the stability of the measurement process. For example, the definition of an analytical run in the first edition (1991) of the Clinical and Laboratory Standards Institute (CLSI) document C24-A, *Internal Quality Control Testing: Principles and Definitions*, is the interval within which the accuracy and precision of the testing system is expected to be stable.[2]

In recent decades, it has become increasingly apparent that these historically established principles are no longer optimal, by themselves, to meet the need for a comprehensive QC protocol for the clinical laboratory. Developments in the technology of measuring systems have produced systems in which the interval within which the accuracy and precision of the testing system is expected to be stable is measured in weeks or even months. Recognition of this change is reflected in the third edition of the C24 guidance on statistical QC, which states that, "for purposes of quality control, the laboratory must consider the stability of the analytical testing process, its susceptibility to problems that may occur, and the risk associated with an undetected error." The definition of analytical run was also revised to: "An analytical run is an interval (ie, period of time or series of measurements) within which the accuracy and precision of the measuring system is expected to be stable; between which events may occur causing the measurement process to be more susceptible (ie, greater risk) to errors that are important to detect."

Today the focus of testing QC samples in the laboratory has shifted from monitoring inherent drift in the measuring system to detecting two fundamental types of events that can be sources of change in system performance. These events are examples of failure modes. The first type of event is routine planned activities that may be associated with changed performance. Examples of such events are calibration, first use of a new reagent lot, certain maintenance procedures, and system repairs. Each of these events provides an opportunity for change in the measuring system. System performance should be verified around each event.

The second type of event that can alter system performance is random failure of some part of the measuring system. In general, these are low-frequency events that, being random, cannot be predicted. As a consequence, the expected frequency of these random failures is probably not a good basis for establishing the frequency of checking system performance as part of the QC plan (QCP). The stability of the measuring system is, for many systems, no longer a principal consideration in determining the optimal frequency for checking system performance as part of a QCP.

Instead the focus has shifted to basing the frequency of system checks on reducing the potential risk of reporting a significant number of inaccurate patient results.[3] The principle consideration becomes managing the number of possibly inaccurate patient results that may be released before a random system failure is detected, rather than the expected frequency of the random failure.

As the focus of QC has shifted from principally monitoring the stability of the measuring system to managing the risk of reporting inaccurate patient results, it has become more and more apparent that the traditional assumptions about what constituted QC are no longer adequate and the idea of what is encompassed by a QCP needs to be expanded.

In addition, many measuring systems now, especially devices used in Point of Care environments, have built-in sensors that can detect many system malfunctions and prevent inaccurate results from being reported. As these measuring systems have become more sophisticated in their ability to detect failures in the measurement process, some proponents have argued that testing of traditional QC samples is no longer necessary or needs to be done only on an event-related basis such as starting a new lot of reagent. Regulatory agencies have been under pressure to acknowledge these changes and to provide approved alternatives to the traditional frequency of testing QC samples. It has become clear that the self-monitoring capabilities of newer measuring system designs needs to be incorporated into laboratory QCPs along with the ability to adopt future improvements in self-checking and failure detection built into measuring system design.

In response to these trends, in January 2004 the US agency responsible for the CLIA regulations announced 3 alternative options to the default QC requirement. These options were called Equivalent Quality Control (EQC).[4] These options allowed reduced frequency of testing QC samples depending on:

- How much of the measurement process was monitored by internal device controls or sensors
- Whether the laboratory met other specified criteria
- Whether the laboratory could show stable performance for a specified period of time

These options were criticized by many in the laboratory community and, to discuss the issues raised, the CLSI hosted a meeting on *QC for the Future* in April 2005. At this meeting, many of the issues facing clinical laboratories, as well as trends and issues in QC, were presented and discussed. Following the meeting, CLSI created a committee to develop guidelines for risk-based QC planning in the laboratory. In keeping with the CLSI consensus process, the committee included clinical laboratorians, representatives from in vitro diagnostics (IVD) manufacturers, and representatives from regulatory agencies.

The idea of managing risk is not new to health care or to clinical laboratories. Laboratories have long been involved in identifying potential problems in the process of producing reliable diagnostic information and have actively managed these risks. However, this activity has not traditionally been viewed as part of QC. As the idea of what a QCP includes has expanded, many of these risk management activities can now be incorporated into the overall plan.

After 6 years of effort, the committee developed EP23-A, *Laboratory Quality Control Based on Risk Management*,[5] which was approved and published in October 2011. This document was almost immediately recognized by the Centers for Medicare and Medicaid Services (CMS), the US regulatory authority responsible for the CLIA regulations, as an acceptable approach for developing and documenting an individual QCP for the laboratory.

EP23-A: OVERVIEW

EP23-A is built on the basic principles of risk management that have been used by industry for many years. It directly draws from the literature on risk management and the collective experience of the committee members and other individuals who contributed to its development. In particular, EP23-A draws from ISO 14971, *Application of Risk Management to Medical Devices.*[6]

The intent is to help the laboratory community adapt basic risk management principles used in the IVD industry to develop a QCP that will effectively manage the risks of the testing process in the laboratory. EP23-A is not a comprehensive description and implementation guide of risk management techniques. Instead, it serves as an introduction to how risk management principles can be applied in the clinical laboratory to monitor the testing process and reduce the risk of inaccurate results. To that end, EP23-A explains the concepts used, defines the terms, describes a high-level process for developing a QCP, and provides examples. For laboratorians wishing to learn more about the techniques of risk management as applied to in-vitro diagnostics, the CLSI document EP18-A2, *Risk Management Techniques to Identify and Control Laboratory Error Sources,*[7] is a good resource, as well as the large body of literature that exists on risk management in general.

EP23-A describes the QCP as "a documented strategy to mitigate and prevent errors in testing that describes practices, resources, and sequences of specified activities to control the quality of a particular measuring system or measurement process to ensure intended purposes are met." The QCP primarily focuses on the analytical phase of the testing process, but developing the plan requires review and consideration of preanalytical and postanalytical phases as well. The intent of the QCP is not to replace current QC practices, but to expand the scope of what is included and to focus on managing risk through assessment of process risks and selecting the optimal QC tools to minimize the risks. The development of an EP23-A–based QCP can help the laboratory make the best use of all the available QC tools and document how these tools, used together, effectively manage the risks in the testing process.

DEVELOPING A RISK-BASED QCP

EP23-A describes a process that includes the following steps:

1. Gathering information about the testing process
2. Assessing risk in the process
3. Developing a QCP to mitigate risks
4. Implementing and monitoring the plan

Fig. 1 shows the process for developing a risk-based QCP.

STEP 1: GATHERING INFORMATION ABOUT THE TESTING PROCESS

EP23-A describes several categories of information that need to be collected to develop a QCP. These include:

- Regulatory and accreditation requirements
- Information about the measuring system

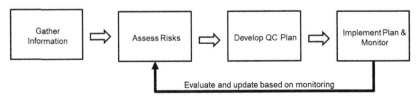

Fig. 1. EP23-A QCP process.

- Information about the laboratory
- Information about the clinical application

Much of the information needed is probably already known to the laboratory and will require little effort to assemble. Some of it may be available, but in a less obvious form, and some information will have to be obtained.

Regulatory and Accreditation Requirements

Any QCP used by the laboratory must comply with all local and national regulations and meet the requirements of any accrediting organizations used by the laboratory, so the laboratory needs to incorporate all these requirements into the plan. Following the EP23-A guidance to develop a risk-based QCP and documenting the process helps the laboratory to provide evidence of regulatory compliance because EP23-A is recognized as an acceptable approach for individual QCPs.

Information About the Measuring System

Information about the measuring system is critical to understanding what possible failures may occur in the system that may lead to reporting inaccurate patient results. Also data and information characterizing the expected normal performance of the measuring system are essential to the effective selection and use of the available QC tools. Information can come from several sources including the laboratory's own experience with the measuring system, or similar systems, and the experience of other laboratories as shared in direct communication or through published articles, peer group data, and so forth.

Key information that may come from the laboratory's experience is the performance characteristics of the measuring system in that specific laboratory environment. Characteristics such as precision, bias, verification of reportable range, and reference interval are all important in the selection and effective use of specific QC tools as part of the development of a QCP. However, especially with systems new to the laboratory, information from the system's manufacturer may be a principle source.

IVD manufacturers use risk management as an integral part of the design and development of their products. Risk assessment is used to identify potential failure modes that may affect product performance or safety. To the degree that is practical, these potential failure modes are mitigated as part of the design and development process. Then risk assessment is applied again to evaluate any residual risks. The results of this risk management process are shared with the laboratory primarily in two forms. First is the design of the analytical system, which mitigates as many potential failure modes as practical. Second is information on how to mitigate any residual risks.

As noted earlier, manufacturers mitigate identified potential failure modes as part of the design and development process. Some of these mitigations are effectively complete with no significant residual risk. An example might be monitoring the temperature of the analytical process and blocking the reporting of any result if the temperature exceeds the limits for an accurate analysis.

For some failure modes, it may not be possible for the manufacturer to incorporate mitigations into the design. These risks typically involve factors outside the manufacturer's control. Most commonly, this occurs when the manufacturer needs to rely on the laboratory to perform certain tasks such as proper storage of reagents, proper preparation of reagents, and correct loading of samples or reagents onto the system. Information about these failure modes and the recommended mitigations are typically included in the product documentation or instructions for use. Key information is found in the instructions for use for individual reagents or consumables as well as for the overall measuring system. EP23-A states: "Manufacturers should provide adequate instructions for use. These instructions typically include the intended use, test procedure, technical performance, maintenance, and storage recommendations (temperature, humidity, and light), environmental conditions of operation, limitations, and other information needed to properly install, verify, and use the measuring system."[5]

Because the product documentation and instructions for use are developed to provide details on safe and effective use of the product, and most were written before EP23-A was published, the information on mitigating potential process failures is not compiled in a single place, but is incorporated throughout the instructions for use where relevant to the use of the product. For a typical instrument system used in the laboratory, there are not only instructions for use of the instrument system itself but also for the reagents, calibrators, QC material, and possibly some other consumables as well. As a consequence, when assembling information about the measuring system, it is necessary to read through all of the relevant instructions for use (system, reagent, consumable, and so forth) and compile the mitigation information. It is hoped that, as the use of risk-based QCPs becomes more widespread in laboratories, manufacturers may facilitate the laboratory's efforts by providing the risk information from the instructions for use already compiled in a format to support development of a QCP.

Another group of identified failure modes may be largely mitigated by design, but may have some residual risk that may need to be accounted for in the QCP. An example might be clot detection for a sampling probe. The technology used may detect most clots, but may not be able to detect very small formed clots or strands of fibrin floating in the serum or plasma. Another example might be an assay or test that is not affected by the presence of small amounts of hemoglobin in the sample, but may be affected by larger concentrations. In these cases, there may be residual risk that needs to be evaluated when developing the QCP. To be able to decide what risk mitigation is needed, the potential impact of the residual risk and the limitations of the design feature need to be understood in more detail. EP23-A states, "Awareness of key risk mitigation features for the measuring system is another important piece of information necessary for development of an appropriate and effective QCP. If a laboratory needs additional information from the manufacturer to develop a QCP, it should contact the manufacturer and request detailed information." In many cases, the information needed is included in the instructions for use. In the example of hemolysis affecting the result, there may be data in the instructions for use showing the impact of hemolysis on results or indicating the maximum acceptable hemoglobin concentration. In other cases, the laboratory may need to contact the manufacturer for additional information.

When contacting the manufacturer, there are a few key things to keep in mind. Just as the development and use of risk-based QCPs is new to the clinical laboratory, this type of laboratory QCP is also new to manufacturers. Although IVD manufacturers have long used risk management in product design control as well as managing product life cycles, the idea of providing laboratories with consolidated information to support development of risk-based QCPs is new and manufacturers need time to develop the best mechanisms and formats to provide the information. Manufacturers should have hazard and failure mode documentation for all their products, but much of the information contained may not be relevant to the development of a risk-based QCP. A risk-based QCP should be focused on identification and management of those failure modes that may lead to the reporting of an inaccurate patient result. The manufacturer's product risk assessment documentation contains more than that. Manufacturers have to address many types of risk when developing products. They have to address safety risks to product users, safety risks to manufacturing staff and field service personnel, maintenance and serviceability hazards, risks to the product during shipment, risks if failure of one part may lead to other hazards, and so forth.

As a consequence, some information requested by the laboratory for use in developing their QCP may not be available on request. One way to facilitate obtaining the information to use for the QCP is to make sure the requested information is specific. A request for all risk information necessary for an EP23-A–based QCP will likely get a response asking for specifics. A better approach is to thoroughly review the existing information in the instructions for use, determine what additional information may be relevant for specific potential failure modes, and then request information not included in the existing documentation. For example, a request for a statement of which measurement methods are sensitive to the presence of small clots or fibrin strands and the minimum clot size that can be detected by the clot detection feature is more specific and may be pertinent to the development of a QCP.

The information available may not be exactly what is requested. For example, the manufacturer may have set a design specification that the clot detection feature should detect clots of a certain size with a probability of 90%. The information available would document that this performance specification is met. There may not be specific information available on whether smaller clots or fibrin strands may also be detected.

Information About the Laboratory

Because the environment around the measuring system and the operators who use it can influence the testing process, information about the laboratory also needs to be included when assessing the overall testing process. Are all environmental requirements that are specified in the manufacturer's instructions for use met? Are there any periodic changes to the laboratory's environment, such as seasonal temperature or humidity changes? What is the potential impact of these changes on the testing process? Is water quality critical to the testing process? How is water quality verified and maintained? How are reagents and other supplies stored? Do storage conditions meet all requirements for the measuring system?

Another factor that needs to be assessed is the operators who use the measuring system. What is their training and competence on all aspects of their roles? Operators may know how to test samples using the measuring system, but what is their skill/ knowledge level for detecting potential problems, for troubleshooting, for awareness of factors that may affect the testing process? Are they capable of performing maintenance, calibration, and so forth? All these considerations need to be taken into account when developing the QCP.

In addition, the frequency of patient sample testing is important to developing a QCP. The frequency of testing affects several aspects of the testing process. First, is the frequency of testing adequate to ensure that operator skills are maintained? Especially for testing processes that include manual steps like dilutions, extractions, calculations, review of results, test system maintenance, and so forth, too low a testing volume may make it difficult to maintain the necessary skill level, and too high a volume may increase the risk of mistakes. The frequency of testing also influences the design of the QCP and how the QC tools are used. For example, in a high-volume laboratory, QC samples may be tested several times over a 24-hour period to optimally manage the risk of reporting inaccurate patient results. Further, monitoring trends in aggregated patient results (for example, average of normals) may be another useful QC tool. In a low-volume environment using the same measurement system, the frequency of testing QC samples may be once in 24 hours to attain a similar level of risk because fewer patient samples are tested, and trending aggregated patient results may not be as useful because there are too few results for this tool to be effective. Also, when testing QC samples at such a low frequency, the stability and handling of the QC material becomes important. It becomes critical to ensure that the QC material is not used beyond its open-vial stability limit and that the QC material is handled carefully according to manufacturer's instructions to prevent deterioration of the QC material being mistaken for process failure.

Information About the Clinical Application

How the test result will be used clinically is a significant factor in the development of a QCP. Is the result used for screening? Diagnosis? Monitoring? Will the test result be used in combination with other test results or clinical information in making medical decisions or will a medical decision be based solely on the single test result? How quickly will the test result be used after reporting? Will the clinician review the result immediately when it is available in a critical care environment or is the result part of a body of information that will be used to make a decision once all the information is compiled and the clinician reviews it all together? This information helps establish the risk of some failure modes and guides what information may be important in developing the QCP.

The final step in gathering information about the measurement process is to create a process map. A process map is a detailed listing or diagram of all the steps involved in the measurement process. In practice, developing the process map may be an iterative process. An initial process map may help determine what information needs to be collected and, once information is collected, it may influence the process map. To be an effective tool, the process map needs to be complete, detailed, and reflect the process being used. There is often a written procedure that is supposed to detail the measurement process, but the actual process used differs from the written procedure. There can be steps that are not considered part of the written procedure because they are common to several procedures. There can be changes that have been made to improve the process, but that are not captured in the written procedure. It is important that the process map reflect the process as performed. In addition, the process map should include preanalytical and postanalytical process steps that may contribute to reporting an inaccurate result. All of the information gathered from the manufacturer, about the laboratory environment and operators, about the frequency of testing, and the clinical application of the test results should be reflected in the process map.

STEP 2: ASSESSING RISK IN THE PROCESS

Once the information is gathered and the process map is complete, then the risk assessment can begin with hazard identification. The process map is reviewed and places in the process where failures can cause inaccurate results to be generated are identified. These points of potential failure are called failure modes. One way to organize the identified failure modes is a graphic representation commonly called a fishbone diagram. An example of a fishbone diagram is given as Fig. 4 in EP23-A,[5] in which each potential failure mode is diagrammed to facilitate risk assessment and development of the QCP.

Once the potential failure modes are identified, any existing mechanism in place to mitigate the risk should be recorded along with some indication of how effective the mitigation is expected to be and whether there is residual risk. This information can be compiled in a table for review. A detailed example of such a table is presented in Appendix B of EP23-A.

Once the potential failure modes are identified and information about each is compiled, risk is assessed by estimating the probability of occurrence of harm and the severity of harm on scales from 1 to 5 for each failure mode. Then risk is evaluated using a risk acceptability matrix, as recommended in ISO 14971 and illustrated in Fig. 3 of an article by JO Westgard elsewhere in this issue. The basic concept is that failure modes with the potential to cause significant harm need to be identified and prioritized for mitigating or reducing their risks. A table of high-risk failure modes and their associated mitigations provides the basis for the QCP. This table should then be reviewed to determine whether the mitigations are adequate to manage risks to an acceptable level. If the residual risk is acceptable, then no further efforts are needed to mitigate beyond those already listed. If the residual risk is unacceptable, an additional action needs to be built into the QCP to further mitigate the risk. Appendix C in EP23-A provides an example of how to document this process.

STEP 3: DEVELOPING A QCP TO MITIGATE RISKS

When all identified failure modes have acceptable residual risk, the QCP is written to incorporate the actions identified as necessary to both detect process failures and manage risk, and this is when the QC toolbox becomes useful.[5] The QC toolbox is the collection of tools or techniques that are available to the clinical laboratory to monitor the measurement process and detect potential failure.[5] The optimal use of these QC tools involves identifying key points in the measurement process for monitoring, such as after calibration or selected maintenance procedures, after a specified number of hours of operation or a specified number of samples tested, and so forth, which constitutes a return to basing the frequency of system checks on reducing the potential risk of reporting a significant number of inaccurate patient results. Once the checkpoints have been identified, then the appropriate QC tool(s) can be selected to use for monitoring. The choice of QC tool depends on the process step being monitored as well as the capability of the tool to detect the potential failure mode and ensure that the established quality goal is maintained. Details concerning many of these tools, their strengths, weaknesses, and how to use them to maintain the desired quality are discussed in EP23-A as well as in articles by D'Orazio & Mansouri, JO Westgard, Armbruster, Carey, Straseski & Strathmann, Jones, Walz & Darcy elsewhere in this issue.

In addition to the monitoring tools, other actions are built into the QCP to proactively manage identified risks. These steps can include training, environmental monitoring, monitoring expiration dates of reagents, and system maintenance. The QCP should be a high-level outline of the steps the laboratory will take on an ongoing basis to prevent measuring system process failures to the degree that is practical, and detect and follow up on the failures that do occur. The details of how to perform the steps listed in the QCP are provided in the laboratory procedure manual. Each step in the QCP should be traceable back to the risk assessment process documentation. In addition, the QCP should be checked against all applicable regulatory requirements and the instructions for use from the manufacturer to verify that the QCP is consistent with these requirements. For measuring systems that offer a menu of analytes that can be tested, a single QCP may suffice for the system to encompass all the analytes measured, or there may be a primary QCP for the system with some analyte-specific additions if necessary. **Box 1** shows a portion of a QCP found in Appendix D of EP23A. More detailed examples are provided in educational materials available from CLSI.[5]

Box 1
Portion of an example QCP

QCP

- Sample receipt
  - Verify label quality and position
  - Verify adequate sample volume
- System operation
  - Perform all required maintenance per recommended schedule
  - Calibrate system per manufacturer's recommendation
  - Analyze both levels of QC material:
    - After each calibration
    - Before using each new lot of reagent
    - After designated maintenance procedures
    - After system service
    - Every 6 hours during normal operation[a]

[a] Testing of QC samples every 6 hours is based on the expected volume of patient samples tested to reduce risk of reporting inaccurate results should a random failure occur.

STEP 4: IMPLEMENTING AND MONITORING THE PLAN

Once the QCP is complete and has been reviewed and approved by the laboratory director, it can be implemented. Once the QCP is implemented, monitoring the plan for effectiveness begins. No QCP can be perfect and all QCPs need to change as measuring systems, the laboratory environment, or the clinical application of the results change. To keep the QCP current and effective requires monitoring and review. The QC process should be audited periodically to see whether the QC tools are performing as expected. This audit includes review of data from testing of QC samples or similar materials to verify that measuring system performance remains stable and within expected limits. It should be verified that all updates, field corrections, and so forth from the manufacturer have been acted on as necessary and, where appropriate, changes have been made to keep the QCP current. In addition, any time a process failure is detected, the QC process should be reviewed to verify that the QC tools in use functioned as expected and to check whether the failure could have been detected earlier. Complaints from clinicians can be a good source of information on QCP performance. Complaints about process issues like turnaround time or timely communication of results can help identify steps in the process that may need improvement. Complaints concerning discordance between laboratory results and the patient's symptoms or diagnosis can be useful in detecting performance problems. All such complaints should be investigated as far as possible. If the investigation shows that the reported result was inaccurate, the measurement process and the QCP should be reviewed for ways to improve the measurement reliability and/or the detection of process errors. A detailed example of an investigation, the subsequent risk assessment, and revisions to the QCP is provided in Appendix E in EP23-A.

SUMMARY

It may seem as though the creation of a QCP is a large project that may take significant time and effort, and that is true. The necessary steps take time and effort on the part of a team to complete:

1. Gathering information about the testing process
2. Assessing risk in the process
3. Developing a QCP to mitigate risks
4. Implementing and monitoring the plan

Laboratories may want to look to third parties to provide a model QCP to help reduce their effort. However, an effective QCP is unique to the laboratory using it and cannot be provided completely by a third party. Manufacturers are often asked by laboratorians to provide detailed QCPs or recommendations on the reasonable assumption that the manufacturer knows the most about the measuring system design and performance. Although manufacturers may be able to provide information and some guidance, they do not have detailed information about the laboratory's environment, staff, or the details of how the results may be used clinically in a particular health care setting. It is the individual laboratory that should determine which combination of QC tools is practical and will provide the best risk management strategy for its environment and needs.

However, the effort is worth it. A well-designed QCP provides the laboratory with confidence that the risks to patient care are adequately mitigated and the ability to show how that was achieved. This ability can help the laboratory meet all regulatory requirements in a way that supports cost-effective, efficient laboratory operation making best use of laboratory resources and the capabilities of the measuring systems. In addition, a risk-based QCP and the supporting documentation may help address laboratory liability when errors do occur.

ACKNOWLEDGMENTS

The author wishes to acknowledge the invaluable assistance of Neil Greenberg in reviewing this article.

REFERENCES

1. CMS- 2226-F: 42 CFR 493 Medicare, Medicaid, and Clinical Laboratory Improvement Amendments (CLIA) Programs; laboratory requirements relating to quality systems and certain personnel qualifications; section 493.1256 (d) (3), page 1038 Oct. 1 2004 edition. Code of Federal Regulations (CFR).
2. CLSI/NCCLS. Statistical Quality Control for Quantitative Measurement Procedures. Approved guideline. CLSI/NCCLS document C24. Wayne (PA): NCCLS; 1991.
3. Parvin CA. Assessing the impact of the frequency of quality control testing on the quality of reported patient results. Clin Chem 2008;54(12):2049–54.
4. CMS publication 7 State Operations Manual, Appendix C, Survey procedures and interpretive comments for laboratories and laboratory services, subpart K tag D5445, section 493.1256. Available at: http://www.cms.gov/Regulations-and-Guidance/Legislation/CLIA/Interpretive_Guidelines_for_Laboratories.html. Accessed October 12, 2012.
5. CLSI. Laboratory Quality Control Based on Risk Management; approved guideline. CLSI document EP23-A. Wayne (PA): Clinical and Laboratory Standards Institute; 2011.

6. ISO. Medical devices – Application of Risk Management to Medical Devices. Geneva (Switzerland): ISO document 14971; 2007.
7. CLSI. Risk Management Techniques to Identify and Control Laboratory Error Sources, approved guideline. CLSI document EP18-A2. Wayne (PA): Clinical and Laboratory Standards Institute; 2009.

Satisfying Regulatory and Accreditation Requirements for Quality Control

Sharon S. Ehrmeyer, PhD, MT(ASCP)

KEYWORDS

- Quality control • Clinical Laboratory Improvement Amendments • Waived testing
- Nonwaived testing • The Joint Commission • College of American Pathologists
- COLA

KEY POINTS

- In the United States, the Clinical Laboratory Improvement Amendments of 1988 (CLIA) regulate all clinical laboratories.
- The CLIA mandates apply to all clinical laboratories and are based on test complexity.
- All nonwaived testing must comply with the CLIA control procedure mandates.
- The equivalent quality control (EQC) option will be replaced with individualized quality control plans (IQCP).
- Many laboratories voluntarily choose to meet CLIA requirements through following the standards of CMS-deemed professional accreditation organizations.

In the United States, the federal government exerts control through public laws that mandate regulation for all laboratory testing regardless of where performed. In 1988, the US Congress passed Public Law 100–578 for the implementation of Clinical Laboratory Improvement Amendments (CLIA) to ensure accuracy, reliability, and timeliness of patient test results.[1] The CLIA regulations that specify quality testing requirements and personnel standards purposely were written to be site neutral.[2] All testing performed for the diagnosis, prevention, or treatment of any disease falls under the scope of CLIA.

The February 28, 1992 *Federal Register* contains the initial testing requirements for test sites to meet the CLIA law and these are based on the complexity or difficulty to perform a test method.[2] The three test complexity categories are (1) waived, (2) moderate, and (3) high. The moderately complex category includes the subcategory of provider-performed microscopy procedures reserved for special tests by clinicians and midlevel practitioners and performed as part of their practice of medicine.[3]

Department of Pathology and Laboratory Medicine, University of Wisconsin School of Medicine and Public Health, 6175, 1300 University Avenue, Madison, WI 53706, USA
E-mail address: ehrmeyer@wisc.edu

Clin Lab Med 33 (2013) 27–40
http://dx.doi.org/10.1016/j.cll.2012.11.007
0272-2712/13/$ – see front matter © 2013 Elsevier Inc. All rights reserved.

labmed.theclinics.com

Although the Food and Drug Administration continues to classify test methods into one of the three complexity categories, the 2003 update of the CLIA regulations combines moderate and high complexity testing requirements into one nonwaived category.[4] All procedure approved by the Food and Drug Administration in the non-waived category now meet the same requirements with the exception of personnel.

CLIA QUALITY CONTROL REQUIREMENTS
Waived Testing

Typically waived methodologies are performed at point of care and include the simplest testing, as defined by CLIA. In 1992, only eight analytes appeared on the waived list; now more than 100 analytes and hundreds of methodologies are included in this category.[5] The CLIA categories for all test methods are available on the Center for Medicare and Medicate Service (CMS) Web site.[6] As for specific waived testing (WT) requirements, none are identified other than to have an appropriate and current CLIA certificate and to follow the manufacturers' instructions, which may or may not specify quality control (QC) practices. Test sites have the option to implement their own more stringent, QC protocols to assess method and instrument performance. CMS inspectors responsible for determining compliance with CLIA standards do not inspect WT unless a specific complaint has been lodged or fraudulent activities are suspected.

Nonwaived Testing

With the 2003 CLIA revisions, the CMS introduced subpart K, quality systems for non-waived testing.[4] This section is organized to follow the path of patient specimens through the testing process (preanalytical, analytical, and postanalytical). The general QC procedures for qualitative and quantitative tests are included in the analytical section (493.1256) and shown in **Table 1**. It should be noted that CLIA excludes "quality" in identifying control procedure requirements. Sections 493.1261 to 493.1276 contain additional QC requirements for specialty areas of testing. CLIA also mandates (§493.1250) test sites "...to monitor and evaluate the overall quality of the analytic systems and correct identified problems...."[4] QC activities must be part of these activities.

The fundamental premise of the CLIA regulations is that test sites must follow, at a minimum, the manufacturer's directions (§493.1256[d][1]). For most quantitative tests, two levels of QC per day is the minimum, general rule for QC frequency (§493.1256[d][3][i]). The laboratory director must determine whether or not this minimum requirement is sufficient to assess the method's performance and ensure that medical needs are met. For some analytes (eg, blood gases) more levels of QC or more frequent QC are required (see §493.1261–§493.1278).

MEETING CLIA'S QC REQUIREMENTS

Test sites generally meet the divergent CLIA QC requirements in §493.1256(a) to (d) (see **Table 1**) for nonwaived testing through the following approaches[7]:

- Default QC: Each day of testing, test sites can meet the minimum (default) requirement (§493.1256[d][3][i]) for most analytes by analyzing at least two levels of controls per 24-hour period of time and judging the acceptability of the method's performance based on the QC rule the site selects.
- Right Statistical QC: CLIA §493.1256(a) to (c) mandate laboratories to have control procedures that monitor the accuracy and precision of the complete analytical process...establish the number, type and frequency of testing control materials used... detect immediate errors that occur due to test system failure,

Table 1
CLIA QC requirements for nonwaived testing

§493.1256	**Standard: Control Procedures**
§493.1256(a)	For each test system, the laboratory is responsible for having control procedures that monitor the accuracy and precision of the complete analytical process.
§493.1256(b)	The laboratory must establish the number, type, and frequency of testing control materials using, if applicable, the performance specifications verified or established by the laboratory as specified in §493.1253(b)(3) [verification of performance specifications].
§493.1256(c)	The control procedures must: 1. Detect immediate errors that occur due to test system failure, adverse environmental conditions, and operator performance. 2. Monitor over time the accuracy and precision of test performance that may be influenced by changes in test system performance and environmental conditions, and variance in operator performance.

§493.1256(d)	Unless CMS approves a procedure, specified in Appendix C of the State Operations Manual [SOM] that provides equivalent quality testing [EQC], the laboratory must:
	1. Perform control procedures as defined [above] unless otherwise specified in the additional specialty and subspecialty requirements at §§493.1261–.1278.
	    [Microbiology (Bacteriology, Mycobacteriology, Mycology, Parasitology, Virology) §§493.1261–.1265; Routine chemistry (Blood gas analyses) §493.1267; Hematology (Manual cell counts; manual and nonmanual coagulation) §493.1269; Immunohematology §493.127; Histopathogy §493.1273; Cytology §493.1274]
	2. For each test system, perform control procedures using the number and frequency specified by the manufacturer or established by the laboratory when they meet or exceed the requirements in paragraph (d)(3) of this section.
	3. At least once each day patient specimens are assayed or examined perform the following for:
	    i. Each quantitative procedure, include two control materials of different concentrations;
	    ii. Each qualitative procedure, include a negative and positive control material;…

§493.1256(d)(7)	Over time, rotate control material testing among all operators who perform the test.
§493.1256(d)(8)	Test control materials in the same manner as patient specimens.
§493.1256(d)(9)	When using calibration material as a control material, use calibration material from a different lot number than that used to establish a cut-off value or to calibrate the test system.

§493.1256(d)(10)	Establish or verify the criteria for acceptability of all control materials.
	    i. When control materials providing quantitative results are used, statistical parameters (for example, mean and standard deviation) for each batch and lot number of control materials must be defined and available.
	    ii. The laboratory may use the stated value of a commercially assayed control material provided the stated value is for the methodology and instrumentation employed by the laboratory and is verified by the laboratory.
	    iii. Statistical parameters for unassayed control materials must be established over time by the laboratory through concurrent testing of control materials having previously determined statistical parameters.

(continued on next page)

Table 1 (continued)	
§493.1256(f)	Results of control materials must meet the laboratory's and, as applicable, the manufacturer's test system criteria for acceptability before reporting patient test results.
§493.1256(g)	The laboratory must document all control procedures performed.
§493.1256(h)	If control materials are not available, the laboratory must have an alternative mechanism to detect immediate errors and monitor test system performance over time. The performance of alternative control procedures must be documented.

adverse environmental conditions, and operator performance control procedures ... monitor over time the accuracy and precision of test performance that may be influenced by changes...[4] The best approach to meeting these mandates is to select the right statistical QC rules for each analyte based on three criteria: the method's accuracy and precision and a specified analytical quality goal.[8] There are many resources available, including computer programs, to facilitate the selection of the appropriate rules based on actual instrument performance and quality goal information.[9,10]

- Alternative QC and equivalent QC: In 2003 equivalent quality testing, now known as equivalent quality control (EQC), was introduced in CLIA §493.1256(d).[4] Conceptually, it empowers manufacturers to integrate control procedures or systems into the testing device to carry out a variety of quality assessment functions independent of the analyst. Testing devices incorporating this approach are used primarily at the point of care and the assessments are based on electronic, procedural, or internal built-in controls plus a variety of internal function checks. Although not mentioned in CLIA, the CMS considers liquid, external control materials analyzed by testing personnel as the gold control procedure standard. Test sites wanting to meet CLIA's QC requirements with an alternative manufacturer's procedure first must prove equivalency between that approach and the CMS gold standard. CMS in the *Interpretive Guidelines* has specified three EQC options (**Table 2**) to prove equivalency and these are further described in CMS publications.[11,12] To determine which EQC evaluation option to follow, the laboratory determines whether or not the manufacturer's alternative control procedure monitors all, part, or none of the analytical testing process. Based on this decision, the laboratory then conducts the evaluation study lasting for 10 days (option 1); 30 days (option 2); or 60 days (option 3). Option 3 for testing devices with no built-in QC is rarely, if ever, used.

These evaluation studies consist of analyzing external, liquid controls in parallel with the assessments automatically performed by the test device. The collected data from external QC materials and the manufacturer's built-in approach are compared to determine whether or not equivalent information is provided by both approaches. If the laboratory director concludes that both approaches provide equivalent QC information, then the manufacturer's approach, now termed EQC, can be used to meet CLIA's daily control procedure requirement. When EQC is used solely to meet CLIA requirements, external liquid QC must be run periodically to check on the ongoing quality of the device. Periodic assessment is dependent on the evaluation option chosen by the testing site. Options 2 and 3 require an evaluation with external liquid

Table 2 CLIA EQC evaluation options			
EQC Option	Manufacturer's Built-in Assessment of the Analytical Process Components	Length of Evaluation Study	External, Liquid QC Assessment
Option 1	Monitors all of the analytical process	10 consecutive days of testing	Every 30 days
Option 2	Monitors some of the analytical process	30 consecutive days of testing	Every 7 days
Option 3	Monitors none (test system with no internal monitoring) of the analytical process	60 consecutive days of testing	Every 7 days

QC every 7 days and option 1 requires an evaluation every 30 days. External liquid QC also needs to be run to evaluate new lot numbers of reagents, new shipments of reagents, and so forth. Test sites must adhere to specific CMS directives for unacceptable EQC or external control results during and after the evaluation process and when various quality assessment activities (personnel competency, PT, and so forth) indicate problems with test quality.[12]

FUTURE OF EQC

It is fair to say that CMS' equivalent quality testing (EQC) approach to meet the daily CLIA QC requirements was controversial from the beginning.[13,14] Many laboratory professionals thought the equivalency evaluation options were unscientific and not sufficiently robust to truly judge the ability of the manufacturers alternative control procedures to detect errors. At the 2005 CMS and Clinical and Laboratory Science Institute forum, where representatives from government, professional accreditation organizations, manufacturers, and accrediting agencies gathered to address QC issues, the director of the CLIA program admitted that "CMS blew it" with its EQC approach.[13] To justify EQC, two Clinical and Laboratory Standards Institute (CLSI) committees were formed and charged with "quickly" developing guidelines for manufacturers to describe the capabilities of their alternative control procedures and for laboratories to evaluate the information to implement these approaches. The manufacturer document was abandoned by CLSI in 2010. The CLSI Evaluation Protocol (EP23-A) guideline, Laboratory Quality Control Based on Risk Management, was released in October 2011.[15]

EP23-A explains how risk management concepts routinely used in manufacturing can be applied by clinical laboratories. The outcome of the risk management process is a QC plan (QCP) that describes the specific control procedures implemented to ensure quality test results are generated for the circumstances of the test site. The development process begins with gathering medical, regulatory, and accreditation requirements and information about the test system and health care and test site setting. Based on this information, a risk assessment is conducted so that a customized QCP appropriate for a particular testing situation can be developed. An important component of each QCP is an ongoing assessment for effectiveness to identify areas for improvement as appropriate. To assist laboratories in the QCP development process, two companion CLSI documents containing examples and worksheets are available.[16,17]

At this time, it is not known exactly what or when risk management concepts presented in EP23-A will be incorporated by CMS into the CLIA requirements. It is clear, however, that risk management will play a very important role in future QC/QA activities of laboratories.[13] Two CMS memos written to state survey agency directors and the CMS Web site give clues.[18–20] The March 12, 2012 memorandum summary states[19]:

- ...CMS is incorporating into the Interpretive Guidelines (IG), based on 42 CFR 493.1250, key concepts and graphics from ... EP23...as alternative ... CLIA Quality Control (QC) policy.
- The new CLIA QC policy will be entitled: Individualized Quality Control Plan (IQCP).
- ... IQCPs are a formal representation and compilation of many things laboratories currently do for quality which are already included in CLIA... [and] permits the laboratory to customize its QC plan (QCP) according to environment, reagents, testing personnel, specimens, and test system, as long as the QCP provides equivalent quality testing.
- IQCP will be voluntary: Laboratories will have two choices for QC compliance: 1) Default [external] QC requirement, which will continue to be two levels of QC per day [42 CFR §493.1256(d)(3)]; or, 2) IQCP. Regardless of the option chosen, the instructions and recommendations in the package insert must continue to be met.
- Equivalent Quality Control (EQC) will be phased out: At the end of the education and transition period, EQC will no longer be an acceptable QC option. After the end date, laboratories found not to be in compliance will be cited accordingly. There will be no grandfathering of existing test systems using EQC.

The November 2011 CMS memorandum stated that quality plans based on risk management concepts will be voluntary for professional accrediting organizations and CLIA-exempt states.[18]

Once the updated Interpretive Guidelines are published, CMS should announce a start and end date for the education and transition period for implementing individualized QCPs (IQCP), the term CMS uses to describe the control plan for the entire testing process. The IQCP includes a QCP for the analytical phases of testing. Test sites currently using EQC solely to meet CLIA's QC requirements may continue to do so during the transition period, which typically is a minimum of 2 years.

Essential for all quality plans is an ongoing evaluation component to assess for effectiveness and identify opportunities for continuous quality improvement.[21] A logical monitor to evaluate the analytical component is proficiency testing (PT) performance. Under CLIA, regulatory PT plays a key role in assessing internal quality for nonwaived testing and successful PT participation in a CMS-approved program is a requirement for maintaining CLIA certification.[4,22] **Table 3** lists the CLIA selected or "regulated" analytes by specialty/subspecialty of testing along with the CLIA specified acceptable performance limits (target value ± acceptable limit) for each analyte. Acceptable analyte performance in one PT event consisting of five samples per analyte is at least 80% correct results. A second rule covers all the results in a specialty/subspecialty of testing for each PT event. Acceptable performance is a minimum of 80% correct responses over all analytes in a particular specialty or subspecialty of testing. This rule is rarely violated. Testing sites failing the same analyte in two of three consecutive PT events can be subject to sanctions ranging from being

Table 3
CLIA '88 analytical quality requirements

Test or Analyte	Acceptable Performance
Routine chemistry	
Alanine aminotransferase	Target value $\pm$ 20%
Albumin	Target value $\pm$ 10%
Alkaline phosphatase	Target value $\pm$ 30%
Amylase	Target value $\pm$ 30%
Aspartate aminotransferase	Target value $\pm$ 20%
Bilirubin, total	Target value $\pm$ 0.4 mg/dL or $\pm$ 20% (greater)
Blood gas P_{O_2}	Target value $\pm$ 3 SD
Blood gas P_{CO_2}	Target value $\pm$ 5 mm Hg or $\pm$ 8% (greater)
Blood gas pH	Target value $\pm$ 0.04
Calcium, total	Target value $\pm$ 1 mg/dL
Chloride	Target value $\pm$ 5%
Cholesterol, total	Target value $\pm$ 10%
Cholesterol, high-density lipoprotein	Target value $\pm$ 30%
Creatine kinase	Target value $\pm$ 30%
Creatine kinase isoenzymes	MB elevated (present or absent) or target value $\pm$ 3 SD
Creatinine	Target value $\pm$ 0.3 mg/dL or $\pm$ 15% (greater)
Glucose	Target value $\pm$ 6 mg/dL or $\pm$ 10% (greater)
Iron, total	Target value $\pm$ 20%
Lactate dehydrogenase (LDH)	Target value $\pm$ 20%
LDH isoenzymes	LDH1/LDH2 ($\pm$) or target value $\pm$ 30%
Magnesium	Target value $\pm$ 25%
Potassium	Target value $\pm$ 0.5 mmol/L
Sodium	Target value $\pm$ 4 mmol/L
Total protein	Target value $\pm$ 10%
Triglycerides	Target value $\pm$ 25%
Urea nitrogen	Target value $\pm$ 2 mg/dL or $\pm$ 9% (greater)
Uric acid	Target value $\pm$ 17%
Toxicology	
Alcohol, blood	Target value $\pm$ 25%
Blood lead	Target value $\pm$ 10% or $\pm$ 4 μg/dL (greater)
Carbamazepine	Target value $\pm$ 25%
Digoxin	Target value $\pm$ 20% or 0.2 ng/mL (greater)
Ethosuximide	Target value $\pm$ 20%
Gentamicin	Target value $\pm$ 25%
Lithium	Target value $\pm$ 0.3 mmol/L or $\pm$ 20% (greater)
Phenobarbital	Target value $\pm$ 20%
Phenytoin	Target value $\pm$ 25%
Primidone	Target value $\pm$ 25%
Procainamide (and metabolite)	Target value $\pm$ 25%
Quinidine	Target value $\pm$ 25%
Theophylline	Target value $\pm$ 25%
Tobramycin	Target value $\pm$ 25%
Valproic acid	Target value $\pm$ 25%

(*continued on next page*)

Test or Analyte	Acceptable Performance

Table 3
(continued)

Hematology

Test or Analyte	Acceptable Performance
Cell identification	90% or greater consensus on identification
White cell differential	Target ± 3 SD based on percentage of different types of white cells
Erythrocyte count	Target ± 6%
Hematocrit	Target ± 6%
Hemoglobin	Target ± 7%
Leukocyte count	Target ± 15%
Platelet count	Target ± 25%
Fibrinogen	Target ± 20%
Partial thromboplastin time	Target ± 15%
Prothrombin time	Target ± 15%
Endocrinology	
Cortisol	Target value ± 25%
Free thyroxine	Target value ± 3 SD
Human chorionic gonadotropin	Target value ± 3 SD or (positive or negative)
T_3 uptake	Target value ± 3 SD by method
Triiodothyronine	Target value ± 3 SD
Thyroid-stimulating hormone	Target value ± 3 SD
Thyroxine	Target value ± 20% or 1.0 mcg/dL (greater)
General immunology	
α_1-Antitrypsin	Target value ± 3 SD
Alpha fetoprotein	Target value ± 3 SD
Antinuclear antibody	Target value ± 2 dilution or (pos. or neg.)
Antistreptolysin O	Target value ± 2 dilution or (pos. or neg.)
Anti-HIV	Reactive or nonreactive
Complement C3	Target value ± 3 SD
Complement C4	Target value ± 3 SD
Hepatitis (HBsAg, anti-HBc, HBeAg)	Reactive (positive) or nonreactive (negative)
IgA	Target value ± 3 SD
IgE	Target value ± 3 SD
IgG	Target value ± 25%
IgM	Target value ± 3 SD
Infectious mononucleosis	Target value ± 2 dilution or (pos. or neg.)
Rheumatoid factor	Target value ± 2 dilution or (pos. or neg.)
Rubella	Target value ± 2 dilution or (pos. or neg.)

Analytical quality requirements have been defined by the CLIA-88 proficiency testing criteria for acceptable performance. These criteria are presented in three different ways:
- As absolute concentration limits (eg, target value ± 1 mg/dL for calcium)
- As a percentage (eg, target value ± 10% for albumin, cholesterol, and total protein)
- As the distribution of a survey group (eg, target value ± 3 SD for thyroid-stimulating hormone).
  In a few cases, two sets of limits are given (eg, the glucose requirement is given as the target value ± 6 mg/dL or ± 10% [whichever is greater]).
  Data from US Department of Health and Human Services. Medicare, Medicaid and CLIA Programs: regulations implementing the Clinical Laboratory Improvement Amendments of 1988 (CLIA). Final rule. Fed Regist 1992;57:7002–186.

required to submit a plan of correction to mandatory suspension of testing for the failed analyte.

MEETING QC THROUGH VOLUNTARY ACCREDITATION

The CLIA regulations stipulate that CMS can deem or approve nonprofit, professional organizations having laboratory testing standards that are essentially equivalent to or more stringent than those of CLIA.[2] Although all clinical testing sites must conduct testing under a current CLIA certificate, many testing sites voluntarily choose to meet the CLIA requirements through adhering to the standards of one of the CMS-approved, professional accreditation organizations (AO).[23] Testing sites choosing accreditation must comply with their AO's requirements, pay the necessary fees that are in addition to the CLIA fees, and be inspected by the organization for compliance. In July of 2012, approximately 233,000 testing sites were CLIA certified and 7% of these sites were accredited by CLIA-deemed organizations.[24] The three principal AOs are The Joint Commission, the Laboratory Accreditation Program of the College of American Pathologists (LAP-CAP), and COLA (formerly the Commission on Office Laboratory Accreditation).[25–27] When testing sites meet their AO's requirements, as assessed through inspection every 2 years, the test sites are considered to be in compliance with the CLIA requirements. CMS does retain the right to reinspect a small percentage of these testing sites as a quality assessment check.

THE JOINT COMMISSION

The Joint Commission accredited test sites need to adhere, at minimum, to the waived and nonwaived standards identified in the latest *Comprehensive Accreditation Manual for Laboratories and Point-of-Care Testing*.[25] Unlike CLIA, The Joint Commission not

Table 4
The Joint Commission quality system assessment (QC) requirements for nonwaived testing

Quality System Assessment Number	Quality System Assessment Requirement
02.04.01	The laboratory evaluates (for 10 or 30 days) instrument-based testing with electronic or internal systems before using them for routine QC.
02.05.01	The laboratory evaluates noninstrument-based testing with internal QC systems before using them for routine QC.
02.06.01	Each laboratory specialty and subspecialty has a QC policy.
02.07.01	The laboratory has its own QC ranges with valid statistical measurements for each procedure.
02.09.01	The laboratory performs QC testing in the same manner as it performs patient testing.
02.10.01	The laboratory performs QC testing to monitor the accuracy and precision of the analytic process. Note: This standard is considered in combination with the specialty and subspecialty requirements found in this article (eg, blood gas testing requires three levels of QC materials each day of patient testing).
02.11.01	The laboratory conducts surveillance of patient results and related records as part of its QC program.
02.12.01	The laboratory investigates and takes corrective action for deficiencies identified through QC surveillance.

only requires test sites performing WT to follow manufacturers' protocols, but also to follow a series of specific WT requirements. WT.04.01.01 focuses on QC and states that the organization performs quality control checks for WT on each procedure. Inspectors ascertain a test site's compliance with this and other requirements by using the associated Elements of Performance (EP) for guidance. For WT.04.01.01 the EPs are:

EP-2: The documented QC rationale for WT is based on how the test is used, reagent stability, manufacturers' recommendations, the organization's experience with the test, and currently accepted guidelines.

Table 5 LAP-CAP (QC) requirements for waived and nonwaived testing. Point of care testing (POC) checklist	
Waived Standard	**Waived Requirement**
0.07037	Documented QC results - Controls are documented for quantitative and qualitative tests, as applicable.
0.07124	There is evidence of corrective action when control results exceed defined acceptability limits.
0.07211	The results of controls are verified for acceptability before reporting results.
Nonwaived Standard	**Nonwaived Requirement**
0.07300	Daily QC - Controls are run daily for quantitative and qualitative tests. NOTE 1: Except for tests meeting the criteria in Note 2, below, daily external controls must be run as follows: 1. For quantitative tests, 2 controls at 2 different concentrations must be run daily or with each batch of samples/reagents, except for coagulation tests (2 controls required every 8 h), or unless otherwise required elsewhere in this checklist. 2. For qualitative tests, a negative control and a positive control (when available) must be run daily. Control testing is not necessary on days when patient testing is not performed. NOTE 2: Daily controls may be limited to electronic/procedural/built-in (eg, internal, including built-in liquid) controls for tests meeting the following criteria: 1. For quantitative tests, the test system includes 2 levels of electronic/procedural/built-in internal controls that are run daily 2. For qualitative tests, the test system includes an electronic/procedural/built-in internal control run daily 3. The system is FDA-cleared or approved, and not modified by the laboratory 4. The system is not classified as highly complex under CLIA 5. The laboratory has performed studies (20 days for initial device) to validate the adequacy of limiting daily QC to the electronic/procedural/built-in controls.
0.07428	QC data are evaluated daily to detect instrument or process failure.
0.07456	Acceptable limits are defined for control procedures.
0.07484	There is documentation of corrective action when QC results exceed defined acceptability limits.
0.07512	QC specimens are tested in same manner and by same personnel as patient samples.
0.07540	The results of controls are verified for acceptability before reporting results.

EP-3: For non–instrument-based WT, QC checks are performed at the frequency and number of levels recommended by the manufacturer and as defined by the organization's policies. If these elements are not defined by the manufacturer, the laboratory defines the frequency and number of levels for quality control.

EP-4: For instrument-based WT, QC checks are performed on each instrument used for patient testing per manufacturers' instructions.

Table 6	
COLA QC requirements for nonwaived testing	
COLA Standard	**COLA QC Requirement**
VER (Verification) 12	Laboratory determines appropriate calibration and QC frequencies based on the test system's performance specifications.
QC 1	QC program monitors the complete analytic process for each test performed.
QC 2–QC 6	QC program defines: QC 2: The frequency of performing controls. QC 3: The number of controls to perform. QC 4: The type of controls to perform. QC 5: The acceptable limits for control results. QC 6: The corrective actions to take if controls exceed limits.
QC 7	Appropriate reference materials are used for controls.
QC 8	Materials used as controls are verified by repetitive testing to meet the manufacturer's established parameters for mean and standard deviation.
QC 9	For un-assayed controls, control values are established by doing concurrent testing with samples of known values.
QC 10	Manufacturer's instructions are followed for the use of reagents, controls, and kits.
QC 12	Controls are run in the same manner as patient specimens and rotated among all operators who perform the test.
QC 13	When QC or calibration material is used to establish a cut off value for determining positive or negative reactivity in patient samples, the test is controlled using materials of a different lot number than those used to establish the cut off value.
QC 14	Controls are run before resuming patient testing, when there is a complete change of reagents, major preventative maintenance is performed, or any critical part replaced that may influence test performance.
QC 15	For quantitative tests, two different control concentrations are performed each day of patient testing.
QC 16	For each quantitative test performed, QC data prepared and plotted with each testing event, or statistical indices are calculated to permit the laboratory to assess continued accuracy and precision of the method.
QC 17	If one performs qualitative tests, are positive and negative controls performed each day of patient testing.
QC 24	Equivalent Quality Control Option: … laboratories may continue to do 2 levels of external QC for each day of patient testing…[they]may elect for eligible test systems that have successfully completed a qualification procedure…[10 or 30 d for alternative QC].

EP-5: For instrument-based WT, QC checks require two levels of control, if commercially available.

The Joint Commission identifies general quality system assessment requirements for nonwaived testing (**Table 4**) and additional QC requirements for specialty areas of testing.

THE LABORATORY ACCREDITATION PROGRAM OF THE COLLEGE OF AMERICAN PATHOLOGISTS

LAP-CAP identifies its testing requirements in a series of checklists.[26] All test sites follow the All Common and Laboratory General checklists in addition to checklists for each testing discipline. LAP-CAP–accredited sites performing WT follow a series of requirements in the Point of Care Testing checklist and these include QC mandates (**Table 5**); compliance is determined through the biannual inspections. Nonwaived testing QC requirements are included in the discipline-specific checklists. The non-waived QC requirements in the Point of Care checklist represent the general QC requirements for all disciplines (summarized in **Table 5**).

COLA

COLA initially focused on accrediting testing performed in physician office laboratories. Now COLA accredits all test site locations, including those in hospitals and other health care organizations. The testing requirements are identified in the *COLA Accreditation Criteria* manual.[27] COLA's QC requirements generally follow the CLIA regulations. Like CLIA, COLA does not have specific requirements for WT other than to follow the manufacturer's directions and COLA does not inspect WT during its biannual inspections. **Table 6** summarizes COLA's nonwaived QC requirements.

SUMMARY

The minimum QC requirements for all US clinical laboratories are specified in the CLIA regulations. The QC mandates are based on test complexity, waived and nonwaived. The only requirement for WT, the simplest level of testing, is to follow the manufacturers' directions, which may or may not include QC directives. The QC requirements for nonwaived testing are included in subpart K, §493.1256, of CLIA 2003. Although this section states that the control procedures must detect immediate errors caused by test system failure, adverse environmental conditions, and operator performance and monitor over time the accuracy and precision of test performance that may be influences by a variety of changes, CMS allows several approaches to meeting the daily QC requirements. The general minimum or default QC requirement for quantitative nonwaived testing is two levels of external control materials per test per day of testing (§493.1256[d][3][i]). Specialty and subspecialty areas of testing may have additional QC requirements. In 2003, CLIA introduced equivalent quality testing or EQC to allow test sites using manufacturers alternate (built-in) control procedures to meet CLIA's QC requirements. From the start, EQC was controversial and CMS in cooperation with CLSI sought to resolve the issues. After the release of CLSI's guideline, EP23-A, CMS announced that EQC as a sole means to meet the CLIA QC requirements will be phased out and replaced by individualized QCPs, based on risk management concepts to be included in the updated CMS Interpretive Guidelines. At this time, CMS has not published these guidelines or announced the start and end date of the education and transition period for implementing IQCPs that address the entire testing process and contain control procedures for the analytical phase of testing and an assessment component to evaluate overall effectiveness and identify opportunities for improvement. Although CMS sets the minimum US testing requirements, many clinical laboratories choose to meet these through complying with the testing standards of a CMS "deemed" or approved professional AO.

REFERENCES

1. Pub L No. 100-578, §353, Publish Health Service Act of 1988, 42 USC §263a. Available at: http://wwwn.cdc.gov/clia/pdf/PHSA_353.pdf. Accessed September 17, 2012.
2. US Department of Health and Human Services. Medicare, Medicaid and CLIA programs: regulations implementing the Clinical Laboratory Improvement Amendments of 1988 (CLIA). Final rule. Fed Regist 1992;57:7002–186.
3. Provider-performed microscopy procedures. Available at: http://www.cms.gov/Regulations-and-Guidance/Legislation/CLIA/Downloads/ppmplist.pdf. Accessed September 17, 2012.
4. US Centers for Medicare, Medicaid Services (CMS). Medicare, Medicaid, and CLIA programs: laboratory requirements relating to quality systems and certain personnel qualifications. Final rule. Current CLIA regulations (including all changes through 01/24/2003). Fed Regist 2003;16:3640–714. Available at: http://wwwn.cdc.gov/clia/regs/toc.aspx. Accessed September 17, 2012.
5. Tests granted waived status under CLIA. Available at: http://www.cms.gov/Regulations-and-Guidance/Legislation/CLIA/Downloads/waivetbl.pdf. Accessed September 17, 2012.
6. Categorization of tests. Available at: http://www.cms.gov/Regulations-and-uidance/Legislation/CLIA/Categorization_of_Tests.htm. Accessed September 17, 2012.
7. Ehrmeyer SS. The new poor lab's guide to the regulations. Madison (WI): Westgard QC, Inc; 2012.
8. Westgard JO. Assuring the right quality right. Madison (WI): Westgard QC, Inc; 2007.
9. Westgard JO. EZ Rules 3 QC design software. Madison (WI): Westgard QC, Inc; 2005.
10. Westgard JO. Basic QC practices. Madison (WI): Westgard QC, Inc; 2010.
11. CMS state operations manual appendix C, survey procedures and interpretive guidelines for laboratories and laboratory services (Subpart K, Part 1). Available at: http://www.cms.gov/Regulations-and-Guidance/Legislation/CLIA/Interpretive_Guidelines_for_Laboratories.html. Accessed September 17, 2012.
12. Clinical Laboratory Improvement Amendments (CLIA). Equivalent Quality Control (EQC) Procedures Brochure #4. Available at: http://www.cms.gov/Regulations-and-Guidance/Legislation/CLIA/Downloads/6066bk.pdf. Accessed September 17, 2012.
13. Malone BA. New approach to quality control? Clin Lab News 2011;37(11). Available at: http://www.aacc.org/publications/cln/2011/november/Pages/ANewApproachto QualityControl.aspx#. Accessed September 17, 2012.
14. Laessig RH, Ehrmeyer SS. We blew it: great partnerships are going to fix it. Lab Med 2005;36(10):577–81.
15. CLSI EP23-A. Laboratory quality control based on risk management. Wayne (PA): Clinical Laboratory Standards Institute; 2011.
16. CLSI. Laboratory quality control based on risk management; workbook. Wayne (PA): Clinical Laboratory Standards Institute; 2011.

17. CLSI. Laboratory quality control based on risk management; worksheet. Wayne (PA): Clinical Laboratory Standards Institute; 2011.

18. Initial plans and policy implementation for Clinical and Laboratory Standards Institute (CLSI) Evaluation Protocol-23 (EP), 'Laboratory Quality Control Based on Risk Management', as Clinical Laboratory Improvement Amendment (CLIA) Quality Control (QC) Policy. Available at: https://www.cms.gov/Medicare/Provider-Enrollment-and-Certification/SurveyCertificationGenInfo/downloads/SCLetter12_03.pdf. Accessed September 17, 2012.

19. Implementing the Individualized Quality Control Plan (IQCP) for Clinical Laboratory Improvement Amendments (CLIA). Available at: http://www.cms.gov/Medicare/Provider-Enrollment-and-Certification/SurveyCertificationGenInfo/Downloads/SCLetter12_20-.pdf. Accessed September 17, 2012.

20. Individualized Quality Control Plan (IQCP). Available at: http://www.cms.gov/Regulations-and-Guidance/Legislation/CLIA/Individualized_Quality_Control_Plan_IQCP.html. Accessed September 17, 2012.

21. Nichols J. Risk management for POCT. Point Care 2011;40(4):139–40.

22. CMS approved PT programs (2012). Available at: http://www.cms.gov/Regulations-and-Guidance/Legislation/CLIA/Downloads/ptlist.pdf. Accessed September 17, 2012.

23. List of approved accrediting organizations under the Clinical Laboratory Improvement Amendments (CLIA). Available at: http://www.cms.gov/Regulations-and-Guidance/Legislation/CLIA/Downloads/AOList.pdf. Accessed September 17, 2012.

24. CLIA update statistics. Available at: http://www.cms.gov/Regulations-and-Guidance/Legislation/CLIA/Downloads/statupda.pdf. Accessed September 17, 2012.

25. Laboratory Accreditation Standards. The Joint Commission. Oakbrook Terrace (IL). Available at: http://www.jointcommission.org. Accessed September 17, 2012.

26. Laboratory Accreditation Program. College of American Pathologists (CAP). Northfield (IL). Available at: http://www.cap.org/apps/cap.portal?_nfpb=true&_pageLabel=accreditation. Accessed September 17, 2012.

27. Accreditation Manual. COLA. Columbia (MD). Available at: http://www.cola.org. Accessed September 17, 2012.

Prioritizing Risk Analysis Quality Control Plans Based on Sigma-metrics

Sten Westgard, MS

KEYWORDS

- Six Sigma • Sigma-metrics • Risk analysis • Risk management
- Failure mode and effects analysis • Quality control design • Quality Control Plan

KEY POINTS

- EP23A empowers the laboratory to choose among many risk assessment techniques to design an individualized quality control plan.
- Failure mode and effects analysis (FMEA), a technique commonly used in risk assessment, has been observed to exhibit key weaknesses in health care implementations.
- Six Sigma is a technique that allows objective assessment of process performance.
- The Sigma-metric quantifies the performance (and thus the risk) of an analytical testing process.
- The method decision chart is a visual tool that differentiates Sigma performance.
- The operating specifications chart is a visual tool that identifies the quality control (QC) required by a test, based on Sigma performance.
- Six Sigma QC design tools can enhance FMEA, the risk assessment process, and design of QC plans.

INTRODUCTION

The new document EP23A "Laboratory Quality Control Based on Risk Management" is poised to make significant changes on quality control (QC) practices in US laboratories. EP23A, a copyrighted guideline from the Clinical Laboratory Standards Institute (CLSI), provides a general description of risk management activities, including a QC toolbox of techniques that can be used to build a QC plan (QCP) to assure the quality of laboratory tests. The EP23A guideline is descriptive, not prescriptive, and the QC toolbox is not meant to be a complete and all-inclusive list of options. While the guideline explains possible choices, it does not require the laboratory to use any specific technique or to follow any specific methodology. This is both a strength and a weakness. Laboratories following the EP23A guideline have the flexibility to use additional

Client Services and Technology, Westgard QC, 7614 Gray Fox Trail, Madison WI 53717, USA
E-mail address: sten@westgard.com

Clin Lab Med 33 (2013) 41–53
http://dx.doi.org/10.1016/j.cll.2012.11.008
0272-2712/13/$ – see front matter © 2013 Elsevier Inc. All rights reserved.
labmed.theclinics.com

techniques and optimizations of existing techniques as part of their QCP. The down side is that laboratories will need to carefully study and examine risk methodologies and techniques before developing QCPs.

WHAT IS A QCP?

One definition states that a QCP is an "optimized balance of control sample analysis combined with manufacturer engineered control processes in the instrument and laboratory implemented control processes to minimize risk of error and harm to a patient when using the instrument for laboratory testing."[1] In 2012, Centers for Medicaid and Medicare Services (CMS) released a promotional brochure touting the benefits of an individualized QCP (IQCP)[2]:

- "Customizes QC plan for each test in its unique environment
- Optimizes use of electronic/integrated controls
- Offers laboratories flexibility in achieving QC compliance
- Adaptable for future advancements in technology
- Incorporates other sources of quality Information
- Strengthens manufacturer/laboratory partnerships
- Formalizes risk management data already maintained within the laboratory
- Provides equivalent quality testing to meet the CLIA (Clinical Laboratory Improvement Amendments) QC regulations"

Clearly, the new IQCP approach builds upon current quality control practices. It is not meant to replace statistical QC, but to augment it by integrating other quality assurance activities performed either by the instrument itself or by the laboratory.

This discussion will focus on additional techniques and tools that can enhance and focus the risk management activities and provide data-driven guidance to QCPs. Six Sigma, a quality management technique popular not only in industry and manufacturing, but also in health care, provides a useful benchmarking scale, easily understood by even the most novice laboratory technician as well as nontechnical staff members who interact with and govern the laboratory's activities.

WHAT IS SIX SIGMA?

Motorola developed the Six Sigma methodology back in the 1980s, as part of an effort to improve the quality of its manufacturing.[3] It was most famously adopted by General Electric, where it was credited with impressive gains in not only quality, but also profitability.[4] The following decades have seen multiple industries adopt Six Sigma methodology, including health care institutions.[5] In health care, Six Sigma applications have been documented in a myriad of processes, for example, catheter use,[6] drug therapy,[7] and analytical testing processes.

Simply put, Six Sigma provides a scale, a benchmark for quality, with the ideal goal of achieving near perfection or almost defect-free operation. The benchmarks are based on the measurement of defects occurring per million outcomes (DPM) of a process. For example, the number of defective results in a million analytical tests could be assessed on the Sigma scale. If the eponymous Six Sigma is actually achieved, only 3.4 defects per 1 million outcomes will occur. If Three Sigma is achieved, however, then the defect rate is close to 67,000 defects per 1 million outcomes. In traditional Six Sigma applications, the goal for process performance is Six Sigma, and Three Sigma is considered the minimum acceptable performance. Outside of health care, in particular, a process below Three Sigma is considered too unreliable for routine operation. A process with more than 67,000 defects per 1 million outcomes would typically be considered an urgent target for improvement, possible redesign, or even replacement.

Nevelainen and colleagues[8] did landmark work focused on Six Sigma assessment of laboratory processes, and found many of them wanting; most of the processes he analyzed were in the Three Sigma to Four Sigma range, and some were below Three Sigma. More recently, the Catalan Health Institute published a multiyear study of its laboratory quality indicators, assessing performance on the Six Sigma scale.[9] While improvements can be seen in those results, particularly in the area of preanalytical performance, the Spanish study showed that analytical performance and the proper use of controls remain chronic problems for most laboratories. A more recent study of the frequency of laboratory errors at the University Hospital of Padua, Italy, confirms that improvements have been made in preanalytical processes, but analytical processes continue to have persistent difficulties (**Figs. 1** and **2**).[10]

Six Sigma can provide a major contribution to risk management of laboratory processes through its measure of quality on the Sigma scale and the benchmarks that aid laboratories in prioritizing the need for improvement of their processes and operations. Six Sigma provides an objective assessment of performance relative to defined quality goals or requirements, together with performance observed for a method, thereby allowing the laboratory to target those processes that are inadequate and in need of corrective action and improvement.

For analytical testing processes, the assessment of quality on the Sigma scale makes use of the known measures of analytic performance in terms of imprecision and bias. Since some amount of variation is present in every test result, one has to be careful about the definition of defect when it relates to laboratory tests. In Six Sigma terms, the outcome of a process is a defect when a test result exceeds the tolerance limits set around the true or expected value. The "Six" in Six Sigma refers to the gap or distance between the true value of a process and those tolerance limits; the goal is to squeeze down the measurement variation of the process until 6 standard deviations (SD) can fit into that space. Why 6? The theory is that even when small process shifts

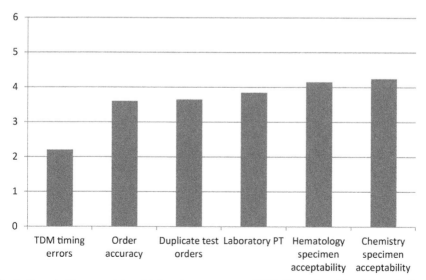

Fig. 1. Sample Sigma-metrics of laboratory processes, 2000. (*Data from* Nevalainen D, Berte L, Kraft C, et al. Evaluating laboratory performance on quality indicators with the Six Sigma scale. Arch Pathol Lab Med 2000;124:518.)

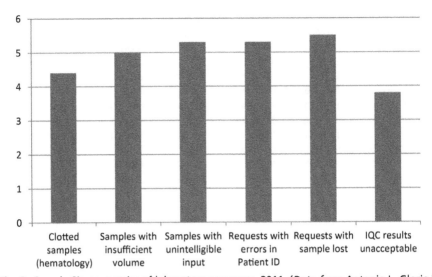

Fig. 2. Sample Sigma-metrics of laboratory processes, 2011. (*Data from* Antonia L, Gloria T, Isabel L, et al. Quality indicators and specifications for key analytical-extraanalytical processes in the laboratory. Five years' experience using the Six Sigma concept. Clin Chem Lab Med 2011;49(3):463–70.)

occur, up to 1.5 times the standard deviation, as part of routine operation, this number of defects produced will still be minimized to just 3.4 per 1 million results.

The short-term Sigma model assumes that up to a 1.5 SD shift may occur during routine operation (**Fig. 3**). Thus, that process must be able to tolerate that amount of variation plus the additional variation of the process.

For laboratory tests, the concept of Six Sigma tolerance limits may sound new. Laboratories are more familiar with the concept of the allowable total error (TEa). When a test result exceeds the TEa, the result is significantly different than the true value of the test result (in other words, a defect). Thus, laboratories that are familiar with different resources that specify TEa (eg, the US CLIA[11] regulations, the German Rilibak[12] rules, the Royal College of Pathologists of Australasia [RCPA] allowable limits of performance,[13] and the specifications for TEa based on within-subject biologic variation[14] [also known as the biologic variation database]) can use those quality requirements as the source of tolerance limits for analytical tests.

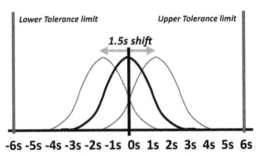

Fig. 3. The concept of Six Sigma. The arrow represents the expected routine variation in a process, which could be as large as 1.5 SD.

HOW CAN SIX SIGMA ACCOUNT FOR INTENDED USE?

According to the CLSI EP23A guidance, "the laboratory should consider the intended medical uses and potential impacts of a patient's test result when creating the QCP... Factors to consider include the influence of the test result on screening, diagnosis, and/or patient management decisions..." Unfortunately, the EP23A methodology never actually considers the analytical quality that is required for clinical use of a test result. Here is where Six Sigma concepts and tools can make a significant impact to assure performance of analytical methods achieves the desired quality and that statistical QC procedures are selected to verify the attainment of the desired quality of test results.

Westgard and colleagues[15] created models or error budgets to judge the acceptability of analytical performance. The first model for total error included bias plus 2 SD. Subsequent models grew increasingly demanding, specifying 3 SD when the demands of proficiency testing were better understood,[16] 4 SD when it was understood that QC procedures were not perfectly sensitive,[17] and finally 6 SD as Six Sigma Quality Management was applied to health care processes.[18] One final significant factor was the vast increase in the volume of testing. In the past, higher error rates may have been acceptable, because the volume of testing was small. Now, however, modern laboratories may generate millions of test results per year or even per month; at that scale, even a 1% error rate causes an unacceptably large number of errors.

Using total error models, it is possible to define the critical systematic error (ΔSE_{crit}): the size of error that is large enough to cause medically important error. Still, the total error models associated with analytical testing need to find common ground with the Six Sigma model. This relationship between Six Sigma and the critical systematic error is established in the following equation (**Fig. 4**)[18]:

$$\Delta SE_{crit} = [(TE_a - Bias)/CV] - 1.65$$

where

ΔSE_{crit} represents the critical systematic error of the test method,
TE_a represents the allowable total error, or quality requirement, for the test method,
Bias represents the observed inaccuracy or trueness of the test method,
CV represents the observed imprecision of the test method, and
1.65 represents the z-value associated with a 5% risk of an incorrect result.

This equation can be restated as:

Sigma-metric = ΔSE_{crit} + 1.65

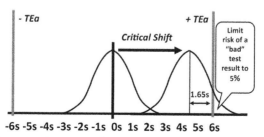

Fig. 4. The critical systematic error and its relationship to the Sigma concept. The arrow represents the critical-systematic error, an error so large it causes a medically important shift in results.

WHAT SIX SIGMA TOOLS ARE APPLICABLE?

Estimation of the Sigma-metric of a laboratory method is useful in itself to understand the real quality that is being achieved by a testing process. But that is only the first step. The next steps are more important: turning that data into insight, practical advice, and action. A graphical method decision chart can be used to provide a visual display of the quality of a laboratory test. With the relationship of the Sigma-metric linked to the critical systematic error, the quality planning tools developed over the past 3 decades can be applied. The most important advice coming out of a Sigma-metric assessment is a recommendation for the statistical QC procedure required for the test method.

The method decision chart uses data on method performance to generate a visual assessment of acceptability. Diagonal lines separate the graph into different Sigma zones. Plotting the method performance with imprecision as the x-coordinate and bias as the y-coordinate allows the user to make a quick visual decision about method acceptability. The ideal zone is near the origin of the graph, where method performance of better than Six Sigma is found, and where very few defects in test results are expected, less than 3.4 defects per 1 million tests. The further a method's plotted point is from the origin, the worse its Sigma-metric, and the more defects are expected in the test results. If a method is performing worse than Two Sigma, that falls in the unacceptable zone; it is expected that the test will generate too many defects to be reliable.

Each chart can be prepared for an individually specified quality requirement (TEa) or a normalized chart can be used, where the method performance is normalized as a fraction of the quality requirement (**Fig. 5**).

Power function graphs describe the probability of rejecting an analytical run versus the size of errors occurring in a run allowing QC performance to be characterized in terms of the probability for error detection (P_{ed}) and the probability of false rejection (P_{fr}) for different control rules and different number of control measurements.[19]

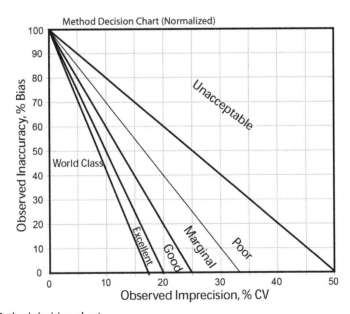

Fig. 5. Method decision chart.

The performance of common QC procedures can be compared so the strengths and weaknesses of different QC rules can be assessed. Critical error graphs apply specific error conditions to those power curves, allowing laboratories to choose QC procedures for any given critical systematic error. The addition of the Sigma scale to the critical error graph is called a Sigma-metrics QC selection graph, and this tool shows the relationship between the Sigma-metric and the critical systematic error. An OPSpecs chart converts the information found in a critical error graph into a graphic tool, allowing simple visual assessment of method performance and selection of the appropriate QC procedure for that method.

In a critical error graph, the critical systematic error, depicted as a vertical straight line, is imposed on a series of power function curves of different QC procedures. The intersection of the critical error line with the QC power curve denotes the error detection capability of that QC procedure to detect the critical error. Ideally, the QC procedure should be able to attain 90% or better error detection of a critical error, which would allow the laboratory to detect the problem almost always in the run when the error first occurs.

The critical error graph imposes a bold vertical line on a power function graph (**Fig. 6**). The power curves in the graph represent different QC procedures. The key details not only the expected false rejection (P_{fr}), but also the expected error detection (P_{ed}) of the critical error.

In an OPSpecs chart, the diagonal lines represent QC procedures that are candidates for use in the laboratory. By plotting an operating point composed of the imprecision (as the x-coordinate) and the inaccuracy (as the y-coordinate), laboratories can visually evaluate which QC procedures provide enough error detection for the method. If 1 of the lines is above and/or to the right of the operating point, that indicates that the QC procedure provides adequate error detection. If there are lines below and/or to the left of the operating point, that indicates that those QC procedures do not provide enough error detection. The OPSpecs chart takes a very quantitative technique and transforms it into a visual judgment, making it an easier tool to use.

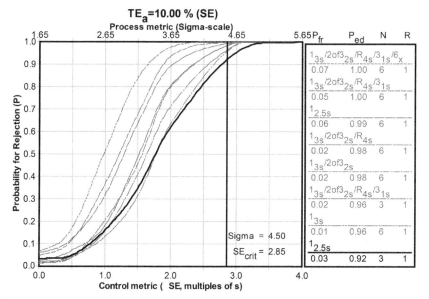

Fig. 6. Critical-error graph.

Although similar to the method decision chart, the diagonal lines in an OPSpecs chart represent different QC procedures, not Sigma zones (**Fig. 7**). As with the method decision chart, the operating point of a method is plotted on the chart, and a visual assessment can be quickly made about the appropriate QC procedure.

DOES RISK MANAGEMENT NEED THESE ADDITIONAL TOOLS?

Risk management, and particularly EP23A's guidelines for development of QCPs, allows the laboratory much flexibility for implementation. EP23A recommends a QC toolbox approach that allows laboratories to pick and choose different tools and techniques, according to their needs and preferences. The drawback to this flexible approach is that laboratories may not know where to start, or what to start with.

An additional concern is the gathering evidence that popular risk assessment techniques may not be foolproof. Failure mode and effects analysis (FMEA) is 1 of the most common techniques used in risk analysis, and while not explicitly endorsed in EP23, the language of the guideline most closely adheres to this technique. FMEA has been widely used in health care, particularly in the United Kingdom, with mixed results.

Shebl, Franklin, and Barber conducted several studies testing the reliability, validity, and accuracy of FMEA risk analysis. They found that different groups studying the same process generated different failure modes, different risk rankings, and different risk mitigation steps.[20,21] In other words, risk analysis by FMEA was not reproducible. Reproducibility is a strong requirement for a regulatory process that every laboratory in the United States may soon perform. If different groups within the same laboratory, or different laboratories under the same conditions, produce different risk analyses, it

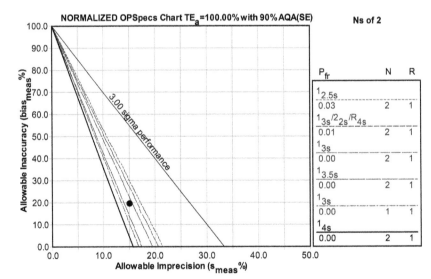

Fig. 7. OPSpecs chart. The black dot is the 'operating point' representing the performance of the method. The x-coordinate of this point is the imprecision. The y-coordinate of this point is the bias. If any of the diagonal lines pass above and to the right of the operating point, those lines represent QC procedures that are appropriate for the method. If any of the diagonal lines pass below and to the left of the operating point, those lines represent QC procedures that do not provide adequate error detection.

will be challenging for accreditation and regulatory agencies to judge the acceptability of their efforts. Furthermore, FMEA required a great deal of time and effort on the part of the health care staff.

Shebl, Franklin, and Barber also conducted numerous interviews with hospital staff in the United Kingdom who had experience implementing risk analysis with FMEA. A few excerpts:

- "The jury's still out on the FMEA process because... has anybody evaluated FMEA as a tool for analyzing risk... When all it is doing is bringing a few things to the surface, which is no bad thing, but it's not a validated process."
- "...Forget FMEA. It doesn't really work effectively, I don't think, and the scores are a hindrance rather than anything else... We wasted a lot of time on FMEA before we realized, this isn't actually working. Yeah, because I think you can get caught up on just the score, that's the thing."
- "The scoring in the FMEA teams need to be the same people, if you change half way through because of the highly subjective interpretation things change dramatically."[22]

Shebl, Franklin and Barber concluded:

"In short, FMEA in health care is associated with a lack of standardisation in how the scoring scales are used and how failures are prioritised. Different team members and different scoring methods yield dissimilar results, and the concept of multiplying ordinal scales to prioritise failures is mathematically flawed. The FMEA process is subjective, but the use of numerical scores gives an unwarranted impression of objectivity and precision. FMEA is therefore a tool for which there is a lack of evidence. It is surprising that such a commonly used and widely promoted technique within health care appears to have no evidence that its outcomes are valid and reliable; particularly as it is used to prioritise patient safety practices and requires so much staff time.[23]

The purpose of EP23A and risk analysis was to provide an easier approach and to determine the amount and frequency of QC, which would help laboratories cope with growing test demand. Risk analysis by FMEA, at least as experienced in the United Kingdom, seems unable to fulfill those promises.

It is important to note that FMEA is not the only tool or technique available for risk analysis. FMEA is not synonymous with risk analysis, nor is it the only technique discussed in EP23A. Given that EP23A identifies many possible tools and techniques, it is reasonable for the laboratory to seek alternatives to FMEA, or adaptions that can improve the performance of risk analysis by FMEA. The addition of Six Sigma, Sigma-metrics, and QC design tools can help ameliorate some of the weaknesses found in the risk analysis recommendations for EP23A.

HOW CAN SIX SIGMA IDENTIFY HIGH AND LOW RISK METHODS?

Although laboratories can use brainstorming, Ishikawa (fish bone) diagrams, and process maps to identify hazards, they can also consult their current data on performance. Using data that are already being collected, a laboratory can quickly leverage its existing quality assurance activities into an objective Sigma-metric assessment. Imprecision is routinely collected on method performance through the use of controls (surrogate samples). Inaccuracy is at least periodically collected through the laboratory's participation in proficiency testing (PT) or external quality assessment (EQA), or more frequently assessed through participation in a peer group program, or initially assessed as part of method validation studies (through the comparison of methods experiment). As mentioned previously, quality requirements in the form of allowable total errors are available from many sources, and can also be defined by the laboratory simply by reviewing the current clinical guidelines on the use and interpretation of the test.

Through Sigma-metrics, it can be easy to identify high-risk and low-risk test methods. Methods with a Sigma-metric of 3 or lower are not performing well, and considering the reduction of QC frequency on these methods will probably only make a bad problem worse. Methods with a Sigma-metric of 6 or higher may be ideal candidates for the consideration of adjustment of QC frequency, because they are performing with very few defects.

HOW CAN SIX SIGMA IMPROVE RISK ASSESSMENT?

If laboratories choose to use techniques like FMEA, the use of Sigma-metrics can be directly incorporated into the risk analysis tools. For example, if FMEA is used with a 2- or 3-factor model, the laboratory may choose to evaluate the resulting risk priority number (RPN) or criticality on a Sigma-scale. Rather than use an arbitrary scale of 1 to 3, 1 to 5, or 1 to 10, the laboratory can use a scale directly built on the evidence of error and defect rates. The resulting risk assessment is more objective, because it is less reliant on subjective rankings, and more reliant on observed performance.

HOW CAN SIX SIGMA IMPROVE RISK MITIGATION?

Even if other risk analysis techniques are used to identify hazards and prioritize risk mitigation, the choice of tools to perform those mitigation activities is still open.

Because detection is the essence of quality control—the detection of errors and prevention of those errors from reaching the clinicians and patients—a strong effort should be made to improve the error detection of QC procedures during risk mitigation. Ironically, the current model suggested by EP23A eliminates entirely the factor of detection, focusing exclusively on occurrence and severity. A vigorous debate exists over whether detection is important in FMEA and risk management.[24] The essence of the antidetection position is that detecting an error once it has happened is too late; mitigation efforts should concentrate on reducing the occurrence of the error and reducing the severity of any error that does occur. The essence of the pro-detection position is that even with reduced risk, there will always be some residual risk that an error will occur. Therefore, the laboratory still needs to have an ability to detect that residual risk, if that error does occur. Laboratories can still focus on occurrence and severity. Detectability, however, is particularly relevant, because the process of QC allows laboratories to detect testing errors, trouble-shoot, and take corrective action, catching and correcting errors before they can leave the laboratory. The Sigma-metric tools and QC design tools allow laboratories to maximize their ability to efficiently, effectively detect those errors.

HOW CAN SIX SIGMA IMPROVE THE ASSESSMENT OF RESIDUAL RISK?

During the risk management process, the assessment of risk and implementation of risk mitigation processes may require multiple iterations. Each time a risk mitigation action is performed, the risk analysis is supposed to be repeated, with a subsequent assessment to determine if the mitigation has lowered the risk of the failure mode to an acceptable level. But for laboratories that are understaffed and overburdened, the pressing question arises, "How good is good enough?" Particularly if risk analysis is conducted with vague, qualitative rankings and subjective guesses as to the severity and occurrence of failure modes, it may be difficult both to significantly change the risk assessment or criticality, as well as assess if the risk has now been reduced to an acceptable level.

The Six Sigma approach can provide a more quantitative estimate of risk, which means that any reduction of risk can also be quantified. The final defect rate can be estimated and placed on the Six Sigma scale, which provides an easy benchmark. If risk mitigation improves a process from Three Sigma to Four Sigma, the number of defects is significantly reduced. Reductions in risk that bring the final process into Three Sigma or higher are a sign that the process may have reached a minimally acceptable level. Reductions in risk that do not bring the Sigma of a process above Three Sigma indicate that performance is still unacceptable, and additional risk mitigation steps are necessary.

AN EXAMPLE: DRIVING RISK MANAGEMENT WITH SIX SIGMA

Recently the EndocLab in Portugal undertook the project to design its QC and QC frequency through Risk Analysis by FMEA and Six Sigma.[25] EndocLab had initially performed Sigma-metrics and used OPSpecs charts to optimize the QC procedures performed for glucose, total cholesterol, and GGT (Gamma-glutamyl Transferase). The results of this analysis determined that these methods were performing at high Sigma levels; thus they were good candidates for further analysis of QC frequency.

FMEA was chosen as the risk analysis technique, and a 3-factor model was used, identifying occurrence, severity, and detection. A novel scale was used for each factor. Instead of a scale of 1 to 3, 4, 5 or even 10, the actual percentages were used, allowing numbers from 0.0 to 1.0 in each factor. This scale was used, so that actual observations in performance could be directly plugged into the factors, so that fewer arbitrary guesses or judgments needed to be used. For example, the rate of occurrence was taken from the frequency of errors reported from the external quality assurance program. The detection factor was supplied by using Sigma-metrics QC selection tool and OPSpecs charts to estimate the probability of error detection for the specific QC procedure used by EndocLab for each method. Finally, the factor of severity was estimated by the laboratory based on its experience of the use of the test results. A ranking of 1 to 10 was used, which was then converted to the scale of 0 to 1.0. The results are shown in **Table 1**.

By multiplying occurrence by severity by detection, one gets a typical risk priority number (RPN). However, one can convert this to a scale of 1 to 1 million. This, of course, is the same scale used by Six Sigma. Thus, one has not only an RPN, but a DPM estimate also. In other words, the residual risk estimate is also the Sigma-metric of the process. One can then quickly assess these methods to see if the residual risk is acceptable.

Table 1
A Risk Assessment of three laboratory tests using FMEA and Sigma-metrics. The resulting Risk Priority Number (RPN) is also the Six Sigma defect rate (Defects Per Million [DPM]).

Test	Occurrence, % QC Errors (OCC)	Severity (SEV)	QC Rules	Detection (DET = 1 - Ped)	DPM	Sigma Short-Term Scale
Glucose	0.86	0.40	Westgard Rules, N = 4	0.08	275	4.9
Total Cholesterol	0.0339	0.60	$1_{2.5s}$, N = 4	0.01	204	5
GGT	0.00001	0.30	$1_{3.5s}$, N = 1	0.10	0.3	6

SUMMARY

As the deadline for abandoning EQC and adopting EP23A looms near, 1 final question arises: is it possible that laboratories are already doing risk management, but just did not know it? Is risk management by any other name still risk management? If the broad concept of risk analysis is simply to improve the outcomes so that possible harm to patients is reduced, the practice of QC has been a risk management tool in use for more than half a century. Proper use of QC, through data-driven tools like Sigma-metrics, is also a risk management technique.

If laboratories choose to adopt EP23A and implement risk management techniques, using established, objective, data-driven techniques will help jump-start that process. Indeed, the use of these techniques is valuable, whether or not laboratories call it risk management, whether or not EP23A is specifically being implemented as a laboratory guideline.

With the cultural obsession for novelty, it is always tempting to embrace the latest "new new thing" and throw out previous tools and procedures. The risk of adopting an untried technique is that useful tools will be abandoned, and steps may go backward, not forward. Building on a foundation of established tools and techniques will help risk management find a better footing in laboratory QC.

REFERENCES

1. Nichols JH. Laboratory quality control based on risk management. Ann Saudi Med 2011;31(3):223–8.
2. CLIA Individualized Quality Control Plan (IQCP) benefits. Available at: http://www1b.cms.gov/Regulations-and-Guidance/Legislation/CLIA/Downloads/IQCPbenefits.pdf. Accessed September 26, 2012.
3. Barry R. The Six Sigma Book for Healthcare. Chicago: Health Administration Press; 2002.
4. Pande PS, Neuman RP, Cabanagh RR. The Six Sigma way: how GE, Motorola, and other top companies are honing their performance. New York: McGraw-Hill; 2000.
5. Harry M, Schroder R. Six Sigma: the breakthrough management strategy revolutionizing the world's top corporations. New York: Doubleday; 2000.
6. Frankel HL, Crede WB, Topal JE, et al. Use of corporate Six Sigma performance-improvement strategies to reduce incidence of catheter-related bloodstream infection in a surgical ICU. J Am Coll Surg 2005;201:349–58.
7. Egan S, Murphy PG, Fennell JP, et al. Using Six Sigma to improve once daily gentamicin dosing and therapeutic drug monitoring performance. BMJ Qual Saf 2012;21:1042–51.
8. Nevalainen D, Berte L, Kraft C, et al. Evaluating laboratory performance on quality indicators with the Six Sigma scale. Arch Pathol Lab Med 2000;124:516–9.
9. Antonia L, Gloria T, Isabel L, et al. Quality Indicators and specifications for key analytical-extraanalytical processes in the laboratory. Five years' experience using the Six Sigma concept. Clin Chem Lab Med 2011;49(3):463–70.
10. Sciacovelli L, Sonntag O, Padoan A, et al. Monitoring quality indicators in laboratory medicine does not automatically result in quality improvement. Clin Chem Lab Med 2012;50(3):463–9.
11. Centers for Medicaid and Medicare. CLIA proficiency testing criteria. Fed Regist 1992;57(40):7002–186.
12. RiliBÄK (Richtlinien der Bundesärztekammer). The term 'RiliBÄK' is an abbreviation meaning literally the Guidelines ("Rili") of the German Federal Medical

Council (BÄK). [in German]. Available at: http://www.westgard.com/rilibak.htm. Accessed October 8, 2012.

13. Allowable limits of performance. Available at: http://www.rcpaqap.com.au/chempath/documents/uploadedfiles/344_GSC%20Revision%20of%20allowable%20limits%20August%202010.pdf. Accessed October 8, 2012.

14. Ricos C, Alvarez V, Cava F, et al. Current databases on biologic variation: pros, cons and progress. Scand J Clin Lab Invest 1999;59:491–500.

15. Westgard JO, Carey RN, Wold S. Criteria for judging precision and accuracy in method development and evaluation. Clin Chem 1974;20:825–33.

16. Ehrmeyer SJ, Laessig RL, Leinweber JE, et al. 1990 Medicare/CLIA final rules for proficiency testing: minimum intralaboratory performance characteristics (CV and bias) needed to pass. Clin Chem 1990;36:1736–40.

17. Westgard JO, Burnett R. Precision requirements for cost-effective operation of analytical processes. Clin Chem 1990;36:1629–32.

18. Westgard JO. Six Sigma quality design and control. 2nd edition. Madison (WI): Westgard QC; 2006.

19. Westgard JO, Groth T, Aronsson T, et al. Performance characteristics of rules for internal quality control: probabilities for false rejection and error detection. Clin Chem 1977;23:1857–67.

20. Shebl NA, Franklin BD, Barber N. Is failure mode and effects analysis reliable? J Patient Saf 2009;5:86–94.

21. Shebl NA, Franklin BD, Barber N. Failure mode and effects analysis: are they valid? BMC Health Serv Res 2012;12:150.

22. Shebl N, Franklin B, Barber N. Failure mode and effects analysis: views of hospital staff in the UK. J Health Serv Res Policy 2012;17(1):37–43.

23. Shebl NA, Franklin BD, Barber N. Failure mode and effects analysis: too little for too much? BMJ Qual Saf 2012;21:607–11.

24. Westgard SA. The detectability debate, June 2011. Available at: http://www.westgard.com/detectability-debate.htm. Accessed September 25, 2012.

25. Westgard SA, Salcedo G. A Six Sigma risk analysis example: defining QC frequency with FMEA. July 2012. Available at: http://www.westgard.com/endoclab-risk.htm. Accessed September 25, 2012.

Analytical Performance Specifications

Relating Laboratory Performance to Quality Required for Intended Clinical Use

Daniel A. Dalenberg, BS[a], Patricia G. Schryver, BS[b],
George G. Klee, MD, PhD[c],*

KEYWORDS

- Analytical performance goals • Analytical bias • Analytical precision
- Roche cobas 8000 • Linearity • Detection limit

KEY POINTS

- Analytical performance specifications are fundamental for evaluating the performance of assays used in clinical medicine and ensuring that they meet clinical needs.
- Analytical goals linked to clinical practice are proposed for 5 performance indicators: precision, trueness, linearity, detection limits, and consistency across instruments and time.
- The Roche cobas 8000 analyzer meets many, but not all, of these goals for 46 chemistry assays.

INTRODUCTION

Analytical performance specifications are fundamental for evaluating the performance of assays used in clinical medicine and ensuring they meet clinical needs. As discussed in the introductory article, manufacturers design their analytical systems to achieve certain performance characteristics for an intended use, then disclose performance claims as part of their information for safety or information for safe use. Design for safety is the manufacturer's priority in mitigating the potential risks of in vitro devices (IVD), according to ISO 14971. In the medical laboratory, risk management should begin with verification or validation that those safety characteristics (reportable

The authors have nothing to disclose.
[a] Department of Laboratory Medicine and Pathology, Mayo Clinic, 200 First Street Southwest, Rochester, MN 55905, USA; [b] Department of Health Sciences Research, Mayo Clinic, 200 First Street Southwest, Rochester, MN 55905, USA; [c] College of Medicine, Mayo Clinic, 200 First Street Southwest, Rochester, MN 55905, USA
* Corresponding author.
E-mail address: klee.george@mayo.edu

range, precision, bias, detection limit, analytical specificity, and reference ranges or cutoff limits) are acceptable for the laboratory's intended use.

These performance specifications should ideally be explicitly defined for each intended use of every specific assay. However, because most tests are used for multiple clinical applications, defining these specifications is an enormous task. Even in well-defined applications it is difficult to define performance specifications that are uniformly accepted by clinicians and laboratory staff because the procedures for defining these parameters are not standardized and there are no consensus criteria for defining acceptable performance.

Middle and Kane[1] recently reviewed the fitness for purpose requirements for estradiol assays. They noted that estradiol measurements have many applications, such as assessment of precocious puberty, infertility, assisted conception, hormone replacement therapy, and estrogen-secreting tumors. They also noted that this test is often interpreted not in isolation but in conjunction with gonadotrophins, prolactin, testosterone, and progesterone. The lower limits for quantification needed for various applications differed substantially. Very low detection limits (<1.0 pmol/L) are needed for assessing children and for evaluating the efficacy of aromatase inhibitors in the treatment of breast cancer. Middle and Kane[1] noted that good precision was important for serial measurements used for assessing infertility and assisted conception. However, even for this single test, the procedures used for establishing these parameters for acceptable performance were not defined and recommendations for most assay performance criteria were not provided.

Multifactorial guidelines have been proposed for the validation of analytical methods. The International Union of Pure and Applied Chemistry published Harmonized Guidelines for Single-Laboratory Validation of Methods of Analysis.[2] These guidelines provide recommendations for the evaluation of 14 method performance characteristics: (1) applicability, (2) selectivity, (3) calibration and linearity, (4) trueness (including reference values for trueness), (5) precision, (6) recovery, (7) range, (8) detection limit, (9) limit of determination or limit of quantification, (10) sensitivity, (11) ruggedness, (12) fitness for purpose, (13) matrix variation, and (14) measurement of uncertainty. The Clinical and Laboratory Standards Institute (CLSI) has developed detailed procedures for evaluating many of the parameters. Each of these validation parameters would ideally have defined performance specifications for each of the multiple applications of each test, but these are seldom available.

This article concentrates on 5 performance characteristics: (1) precision, (2) trueness, (3) linearity, (4) detection limit, and (5) consistency across instruments and time. Each of these performance characteristics has a direct impact on the clinical usefulness of laboratory test results. We have proposed analytical performance goals for each of these 5 quality characteristics for 46 commonly used chemistry tests and have evaluated the performance of the new Roche cobas 8000 analyzer using these goals.

DESCRIPTION OF THESE 5 QUALITY CHARACTERISTICS

Precision is the closeness of agreement between indications or measured quantity values obtained by replicate measurements on the same or similar objects under specified conditions (CLSI EP23A). Precision relates to the minimum detectable differences between serial measurements within an individual or the size of meaningful differences among individuals. Precision performance limits are statistically bound by the magnitude of the biological variation. When the analytical coefficient of variation (CV) is less than 25% of the biological CV, the total CV of the analyte concentrations increases only 3% compared with the biological CV. When the analytical CV is less than 50% of the biological CV, the total CV of the analyte concentrations increases by less than 12%. Analytical performance limits for precision are generally established using data from healthy subjects. Therefore, those precision limits should be applied to measurements in the normal reference range.

Trueness is the closeness of agreement between the average value obtained from a large series of measurements and the true value.[3] Traceability procedures used to define the limits of agreement with the true values are generally based on reference standards or reference methods. Traceability is generally assessed by manufacturers. The European Directive 98/79/EC requires manufactures marketing assays in the European Union to provide traceability of their assays' results to higher metrological orders when standards and/or reference methods exist.[4–6]

A quantitative analytical method is linear when the analyte recovery from a series of sample dilutions is linearly proportional to the target value in the same solutions.[7,8] The College of American Pathologists (CAP) has defined performance limits for their linearity surveys.[9] These performance limits were derived from recommendations for total error limits and are equal to approximately one-half of the allowable total error.[10–13] Analytical linearity is clinically important to ensure that patient specimens with high or low concentrations give consistent results.

Detection limit is the smallest amount or concentration of analyte in the test sample that can be reliably distinguished from zero.[2] There are numerous articles and guidelines about how to reliably measure detection limits, but there are few recommendations for clinically defined performance limits. In general, quantitation of low concentrations is most important for analytes that have decreased concentrations associated with specific disease and/or adverse reactions that can be caused by low concentrations. Almost every analyte has decreased concentrations associated with at least some disorders. Many of these have been enumerated by Young and Friedman.[14]

Consistency across instruments and time is clinically necessary to ensure that laboratory measurements reported to clinicians are reasonably stable. The main issue that systematically affects clinical decisions is a change in analytical bias. This change is similar to the trueness performance; however, there are differences. Consistency is related to multiple single measurements of patient samples rather than the average of multiple replicates of a reference standard used in assessing trueness. There are 3 major causes of changes in assay consistency in clinical laboratories:

1. Differences between multiple instruments used simultaneously
2. Differences caused by changes in instruments or methods
3. Differences associated with changing reagent lots

These differences can be quantitated by regression analyses between the various factors using replicate measurements of patient samples. The bias differences at key decision points can be evaluated using the slope and intercept of the regression lines.

Clinical Performance Limits

Precision
Performance limits for analytical imprecision are generally determined as a fraction of the within-subject biological variability. Fraser and Petersen[15] promoted the concepts of optimum performance defined by an analytical coefficient of variation (CV_A) of less than 0.25 within subject coefficient of variation (CV_I) and desirable performance defined by a CV of less than 0.50 CV_I. This article uses the desirable performance limits for evaluating precision. The imprecision limits listed on the Westgard.com Web site based on the work of Ricos and colleagues[16] are shown in column 5 in **Table 1**.[17]

Table 1
Methods and analytical performance goals for imprecision, trueness, linearity, detection limit, and consistency among instruments and over time

Mod	Assay Name	Units	Calibration Traceability	Imprecision (%)	Trueness (%)	Linearity (%)	Detection Limit	Consistency Low (%)	Consistency High (%)
ISE	Chloride (CL)	mmol/L	Coulometry	0.6	0.5	2.00	77	1.0	1.2
ISE	Potassium (K)	mmol/L	Flame photometry	2.4	1.8	2.50	2.5	2.8	1.9
ISE	Sodium (Na)	mmol/L	Flame photometry	0.4	0.3	1.25	119	1.1	0.7
c701	Alanine aminotransferase (ALT)	U/L	Original IFCC formulation	9.0	12.0	6.25	6.0	25.0	10.0
c701	Albumin (ALB)	g/dL	IRMM BCR470/CRM470 reference material	1.6	1.3	2.50	1.6	1.4	1.0
c701	Alkaline phosphatase (ALKP)	U/L	1983 IFCC standardized method	3.2	6.4	6.25	24	3.8	14.1
c701	Aspartate aminotransferase (AST)	U/L	Original IFCC formulation	6.0	5.4	6.25	8	12.6	6.5
c701	Bicarbonate (CO2)	mmol/L	NIST standard	2.4	1.8	5.00	6	2.3	3.4
c701	Blood urea nitrogen (BUN)	mg/dL	SRM 909b	6.2	5.5	2.50	2.0	16.7	4.8
c701	Calcium (CA)	mg/dL	SRM 909b	1.0	0.8	2.00	6.1	2.8	1.0
c701	Cholesterol (CHOL)	mg/dL	Abell/Kendall method and isotope dilution/MS	2.7	4.0	2.25	62	0.7	1.3
c701	C-Reactive protein (CRP)	mg/L	CRM 470	21.1	21.8	5.00	<0.8	7.8	N/A
c701	Creatinine (CREA)	mg/dL	ID/MS	3.0	4.0	2.50	<0.1	6.3	30.0
c701	Direct bilirubin (DBILI)	mg/dL	Doumas method	18.4	14.2	6.125	<0.1	8.3	N/A
c701	Glucose (GLU)	mg/dL	ID/MS	2.9	2.2	4.00	44	4.6	2.0
c701	High density lipoprotein (HDL)	mg/dL	CDC reference method	3.6	5.2	5.00	9	2.5	2.1
c701	Lactate dehydrogenase (LD)	U/L	Original IFCC formulation	4.3	4.3	5.00	73	3.1	3.3
c701	Magnesium (Mg)	mg/dL	SRM 929 (IDMS)	1.8	1.8	6.25	0.9	2.9	2.2
c701	Phosphorus (PHOS)	mg/dL	NERL primary reference material	4.3	3.2	2.50	0.9	6.0	3.9
c701	Total bilirubin (TBILI)	mg/dL	Doumas Method	11.9	11.4	6.125	<0.1	12.5	30.0

c701	Total protein (TP)	g/dL	SRM 927c	1.4	1.2	2.50	3.6	0.8	1.0
c701	Triglycerides (TG)	mg/dL	ID/MS	10.5	10.7	3.75	28	2.5	5.1
c701	Uric acid (UA)	mg/dL	ID/MS	4.5	4.9	4.25	0.4	6.8	1.6
c502	Amylase (AMY)	U/L	Roche system reagent	4.4	7.4	6.25	4	N/A	N/A
c502	β-Hydroxybutyrate (BOH)	mmol/L	N/A	N/A	N/A	N/A	0	25.0	30.0
c502	Creatine kinase (CK)	U/L	Original IFCC formulation	11.4	11.5	6.25	7	4.6	26.4
c502	Fructosamine (FRUC)	μmol/L	Fructose polylysine standard	1.7	1.7	2.25[a]	153	N/A	N/A
c502	γ-Glutamyltransferase (GGT)	U/L	Original IFCC formulation (2002) and Persijn and van der Slik GGT method (1976)	6.9	10.8	6.25	3	N/A	N/A
c502	Iron (FE)	mcg/dL	SRM 937	13.3	8.8	5.50	6	4.3	3.0
c502	Lipase (LPS)	U/L	Roche system reagent	11.6	10.1	8.75	<10	N/A	N/A
c502	Soluble transferrin receptor (STFR)	mg/L	Roche reference preparation	N/A	N/A	N/A	0.9	N/A	N/A
c502	Transferrin (TRSF)	mg/dL	IRMM BCR470/CRM470 reference material	1.5	1.3	5.00	38	N/A	N/A
e602	C peptide (CPTD)	ng/mL	IRR 84/510	8.3	7.1	10.4[a]	<0.1	N/A	N/A
e602	Creatine kinase MB (CKMB)	ng/mL	Linearized Roche Elecsys CKMB STAT assay	9.9	7.8	6.25	<1.0	7.9	9.4
e602	Digoxin (DIG)	ng/mL	(USP) Digoxin reference material	N/A	N/A	5.00	<0.2	10.0	26.9
e602	Estradiol (ESTS)	pg/mL	ID-GC/MS	9.1	8.3	6.25	<10	N/A	N/A
e602	Free prostate-specific antigen (Free PSA)	ng/mL	WHO Reference Standard 96/668	N/A	N/A	N/A	<0.1	N/A	N/A
e602	Human chorionic gonadotropin (HCG)	U/L	NIBSC 75/589	N/A	N/A	6.25	0	30.0	30.0
e602	Insulin (INS)	μU/mL	NIBSC 66/304	10.6	15.5	16.45[a]	<0.5	N/A	N/A

(continued on next page)

Table 1
(continued)

Mod	Assay Name	Units	Calibration Traceability	Imprecision (%)	Trueness (%)	Linearity (%)	Detection Limit	Consistency Low (%)	High (%)
e602	N-Terminal pro b-type natriuretic peptide (NT-Pro BNP)	pg/mL	Synthetic NT-proBNP reference material	5.0	4.7	6.25	5	8.8	9.9
e602	Parathyroid hormone (PTH)	pg/mL	RIA commercial PTH test	13.0	8.8	15.1[a]	<6.0	N/A	N/A
e602	Progesterone (PROG)	ng/mL	ID-GC/MS	N/A	N/A	6.25	<0.015	N/A	N/A
e602	Prolactin (PRL)	ng/mL	IRP WHO Reference Standard 84/500	11.5	10.5	6.25	<1	N/A	N/A
e602	Prostate-specific antigen (PSA)	ng/mL	Stanford Reference Standard/WHO 96/670	9.1	18.7	4.00	0.1	23.3	25.0
e602	Thyroid-stimulating hormone (TSH)	mU/L	Second IRP WHO Reference Standard 80/558	9.7	7.8	6.25	<0.01	25.8	4.5
e602	Troponin T (TPNT)	ng/mL	Enzymun-Test Troponin T (CARDIAC T) method	15.3	23.7	6.00	<0.01	8.4	23.8

Assays are listed in alphabetical order according to Roche cobas 8000 module.
[a] Linearity limit is 50% or recommended total error limits.

Trueness

Performance limits for analytical accuracy were set at the desirable bias limits defined as less than $0.250 \, (CV_I^2 + CV_A^2)^{\frac{1}{2}}$.[15] The bias limits for evaluating trueness as listed by the Westgard.com Web site based in the work of Ricos and colleagues[16] are shown in column 6 in **Table 1**.

Linearity

Performance limits for dilutional linearity were set at the limits used by the CAP linearity surveys as of October 2012. The CAP performance limits are targeted at approximately one-half of the recommended limit for allowable total error; however, some have been modified to adjust for current state-of-the-art limitations. For analytes not included in CAP linearity surveys, the linearity performance limits were set at 50% of the recommended total error limits. These locally set linearity goals are designated by superscript L in column 7 of **Table 1**.

Detection limit

We estimated the clinically necessary detection limits by examining the test value distributions of large numbers of patients tested at Mayo Clinic Rochester between 2010 and 2011 and setting the recommended detection limits at the 0.10 percentiles. If the percentile was less than the assay reporting limit, the recommended detection limit was listed as less than the lowest reporting limit. However, these detection limits were not evaluated.

Consistency across instruments and time

The limits for the analytical bias across instruments and the limits for bias changes over time caused by instrument and/or reagent changes were set at 1 CV of the changes in the distributions of the test values for the patient population using the technique proposed by Klee and colleagues.[18–20] The logic behind this approach is to keep the systematic laboratory changes in the test values small compared with the total day-to-day changes in the cumulative distributions of the patient test values. Changes in the distributions of the test values may cause changes in clinical decisions, especially for patients having test values near decision points. Although different patients are generally seen each day, when large numbers of patients are considered (such as >1000) the test distributions are often similar. For lower volume tests and/or smaller laboratories, results from multiple days may need to be pooled to collect groups of 1000 test values. The cumulative frequency distributions for 20 consecutive data sets of at least 1000 test values are overlaid and the percentages of test values exceeding key decision points are calculated. Our recommended goal is to keep the systematic analytical bias changes to less than 1 standard deviation (SD) of the observed variations of these cumulative distributions.

Fig. 1 illustrates this technique for albumin, phosphorus, and potassium using the variations of 20 cumulative distributions of greater than 1000 patient test values. The key decision points used for these examples are the lower and upper limits of the reference ranges. The −2 SD and +2 SD limits for each of these decision points are illustrated for 3 tests in **Fig. 1**. One-fourth of the difference between these limits corresponds with 1.0 SD. Our recommended bias limits are calculated as relative percentages at the decision limits. This technique provides multiple bias limits for tests having multiple decision levels. **Fig. 2** shows a cross-plot of these bias limits (on the vertical axis) versus bias limits derived from biological variations (on the horizontal axis). For many tests, these two bias goals are similar, at least at some of the decision levels. We capped the upper recommended limit for the cumulative distribution variations at 30%, because variations greater than 30% were considered excessive.

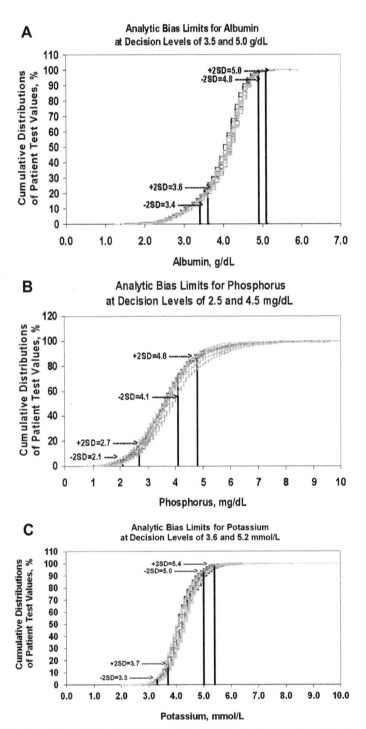

Fig. 1. Variations of cumulative distributions of patient test values used to estimate analytical bias goals for consistency across instruments and time. Examples are shown for (*A*) albumin, (*B*) phosphorus, and (*C*) potassium. The arrows depict the ±2 SD variation at the two decision levels.

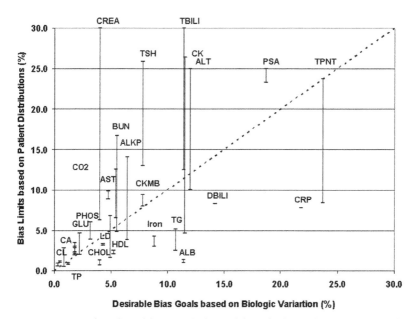

Fig. 2. Comparison of analytical bias goals derived from biological variations, which were used for trueness evaluation, versus bias goals derived from variations in cumulative distributions of patient test values, which were used to evaluate assay consistency among instruments and over time. See **Table 1** for abbreviated test names.

Four analytes had observed values that exceeded 30% because of large variations in the patient populations at some of the decision points (total bilirubin, creatinine, β-hydroxybutyrate, and human chorionic gonadotropin).

Example Applications for Laboratory Test Evaluation

Mayo Clinic Rochester evaluated 2 Roche Diagnostics (Indianapolis, IN) cobas 8000 modular analyzers for placement in the general chemistry area of the institution's high-volume core laboratory where they are replacements for 2 Roche/Hitachi modular analytics systems. The Roche cobas 8000 modular system is designed for high-throughput laboratories, can be connected to the Roche Modular Pre-Analytics system, and can be configured with the core unit, an ion-selective electrode (ISE) module, and up to 4 analytical modules for clinical chemistry and immunoassay testing. The module options consist of a high-throughput (c701) and midthroughput (c502) clinical chemistry modules and an immunoassay module (e602). Each of the 2 Roche cobas 8000 systems evaluated was arranged with a core unit controlling the ISE, c701, c502, and 2 e602s analytical modules. The Roche cobas 8000 test menu evaluation included the 46 analytes shown in **Table 1**. All methods use calibration materials traceable back to the reference methods or reference materials shown in **Table 1**. All reagents, calibrators, and controls used during the evaluation of the Roche cobas 8000 were United States Food and Drug Administration (FDA) approved and used according to the manufacturers' instructions. Roche manufactured reagents were used for all analytes except for Stanbio β-hydroxybutyrate and Genzyme lipase reagents. Samples used during the evaluation of the Roche cobas 8000 systems were deidentified waste serum samples used in accordance with the Mayo Clinic Health Insurance Portability and Accountability Act and the Institutional Review Board policies.

Precision Studies

Interassay and intra-assay imprecisions were assessed using manufactured human serum–based control material and a serum pool. Precision experiments were performed using Bio-Rad Liquichek unassayed chemistry controls on all analytes on ISE, c701, and c502 modules, except C-reactive protein, which used Bio-Rad Liquichek Elevated CRP controls; β-hydroxybutyrate, which used Stanbio β-Hydroxybutyrate/TDM controls; and soluble transferring receptor, which used Roche Diagnostics Tina-quant Soluble Transferrin Receptor controls. Bio-Rad Lyphochek Immunoassay Plus controls were used for precision studies for all analytes on the e602 modules expect for creatine kinase MB and N-terminal pro b-type natriuretic peptide, which used Bio-Rad Liquichek Cardiac Plus LT controls; parathyroid hormone, which used Bio-Rad Liquichek Special Immunoassay controls; and troponin T, which used Roche Diagnostics PreciControl troponin T controls. Quality control material and serum pool concentrations were selected to be within the normal reference range of the assay. Precision studies were performed on the ISE modules, both sample probes of the c701 modules, the c502 modules, and both measuring cells of the e602 modules on each cobas 8000 system. Intra-assay precision was assayed for 20 replicates within a single analytical run. Interassay precision was performed by running both the control material and the serum pool once a day for 20 days. During the interassay precision, aliquots of the serum pool were placed into 20 separate vials and stored at −80°C.

The observed analytical imprecision was estimated by calculating the coefficient of variation (%CV) for both the control material and the serum pool. CVs were compared with the desirable imprecision limits in column 5 of **Table 1**.

Trueness Evaluations

Trueness was assessed using estimates of uncertainty provided by Roche Diagnostics (Indianapolis, IN). The reference methods and reference materials are listed in **Table 1**. This uncertainty (expanded uncertainty; k = 2) was calculated in accordance with the "Guide to the Expression of Uncertainty in Measurement" (GUM: 1993).[21] For the estimation of the single standard uncertainties, normal distribution of the measurement results is assumed. The level of confidence of the expanded uncertainty is about 95%, with the coverage factor k = 2 (analogous to the 2 SD of the standard uncertainty). The percentage uncertainty was calculated by dividing the expanded uncertainty by the calibrator value and multiplying by 100. These relative percentages were compared with the desirable bias limits.

Linearity Assessments

The linearity for each analyte on the Roche Diagnostics cobas 8000 systems was evaluated using Validate GC linearity sets (Main Standards, Windham, ME), Roche CalChek linearity sets (Roche Diagnostics, Indianapolis, IN), or mixing studies of a low and high serum pool. Validate GC linearity sets consisted of ready-to-use 5-level human serum protein–based linearity sets, and Roche's CalChek human serum protein–based linearity sets consisted of either 3 or 5 concentration levels. When Roche CalChek 3 linearity sets were used, concentrations levels 1 and 2 and levels 2 and 3 were mixed in equal parts to obtain intermediate concentrations for a total of 5 levels. When commercial linearity material was not available, low and high serum pools were mixed at 3 parts low to 1 part high, 2 parts low to 2 parts high, and 1 part low to 3 parts high for a total of 5 concentration levels. Roche Soluble Transferrin Receptor calibrator level 5 and saline were also mixed in these ratios because manufactured linearity materials were not available and low and high patient pools could not be created.

Linearity sets and sample pools were analyzed in triplicate on the ISE module, both sample probes of the c701 module, the c502 module, and both measuring cells of the e602 module on each cobas 8000 system. Mean measured values were compared with the assigned or calculated values using least squared linear regression analysis. Slope from the regression analysis was compared with the CAP linearity assessment limits shown in column 7 of **Table 1**.

Detection Limit Evaluations

The manufacturer's stated detection limits are listed in **Table 1**. Some of these limits were locally validated and some were locally redefined. For those analytes locally evaluated, a serum pool at or less than the stated detection limit was analyzed in 4 separate analytical runs over 5 consecutive days for a total of 20 replicates. If the observed %CV was less than 20%, the detection limit was considered acceptable. If the %CV for an analyte was greater than the allowable limit, 2 to 6 additional serum pools with increasing concentration levels were analyzed 4 times a day for 5 days. The mean concentration for each serum pool was plotted versus %CV to determine the concentration at which the assay met the allowable limit.

Assessment of Consistency Across Time and Instruments

Between 50 and 100 serum specimens were analyzed on one of the Roche cobas 8000 systems and on the Roche/Hitachi Modular Analytics system to determine whether these cobas 8000 systems produced equivalent results. The same 50 to 100 specimens were analyzed on the second Roche cobas 8000 system to determine whether the two systems produce equivalent results. Specimens were selected to cover as much of the analytes' analytical measuring ranges as possible and to represent a spectrum of diseases expected during routine use of the method. The specimens were analyzed once on each method within 2 hours and inspected for large differences between methods on the same day on which results were collected. If large differences were noted, the specimen was repeated and reevaluated on the same day on all methods. Up to 10 samples on the ISE, c502, and e602 modules and up to 20 samples on the c701 modules were analyzed on any single day. Testing was conducted over 5 to 10 nonconsecutive days during a 4-week period.

Potential variability encountered caused by calibration or reagent lot changes during routine use was included. The analytes on each Roche cobas 8000 system were calibrated before each analytical run regardless of the manufacturer's recommended frequency. When multiple reagent lots were available from Roche Diagnostics, the reagent lot was changed midway through the experiments.

Method and interinstrument comparisons were analyzed using least squared linear regression. Regression equations were used to calculate observed analytical bias at 2 critical decision levels. The sample range used to determine the linear regression equation was limited to the data around the decision levels for creatine kinase, creatine kinase MB, C-reactive protein, estradiol, iron, γ-glutamyltransferase, human chorionic gonadotropin, insulin, lactate dehydrogenase, lipase, N-terminal pro b-type natriuretic peptide, prostate-specific antigen, parathyroid hormone, troponin T, and thyroid-stimulating hormone to determine a more accurate estimate of analytical bias near the clinical decision points. These analytes had large analytical measuring ranges. Larger differences between methods at the upper end of the range skewed the y-intercept of the regression equation and the calculated analytical bias at low critical decision limits. Method and interinstrument performance were acceptable if the observed analytical bias at each decision limit was less than the allowable limit listed in **Table 1**.

RESULTS FOR EVALUATION OF ROCHE COBAS 8000 ASSAYS RELATIVE TO PERFORMANCE SPECIFICATIONS

The results of the Roche cobas 8000 evaluation for (1) imprecision, (2) trueness, (3) linearity, (4) detection limit, and (5) consistency across instruments and time are provided in **Table 2**. The assays are listed in alphabetical order according to Roche cobas 8000 modules.

Results of Precision Assessments

Intra-assay and interassay precision results using quality control material and serum pools within the normal range are listed in columns 4 and 5 of **Table 2**. The range listed represents the lowest and highest coefficients of variation observed across multiple cobas 8000 modules. If any of the quality control or serum pool precision results exceeded the imprecision limits listed in **Table 1**, they were highlighted in red. On the ISE module, only potassium intra-assay precision was within the desirable imprecision limits. The potassium interassay precision was within the minimum imprecision limit of 3.6% defined by CV_A less than 0.75 CV_I, but chloride and sodium intra-assay and interassay precision were outside the minimum limits of 0.9% and 0.5%. Precision results were within desirable limits on the c701 module for all assays except for albumin, bicarbonate, direct bilirubin, calcium, magnesium, and total protein. Albumin, bicarbonate, and magnesium intra-assay precision were within the minimum precision limits of 2.3%, 3.6%, and 2.7%. Although direct bilirubin interassay precision was within the minimum precision limit of 27.6%, both the intra-assay and interassay precision for calcium were outside the minimum precision limit of 1.4%. Albumin, bicarbonate, magnesium, and total protein were outside the minimum interassay precision limits of 2.3%, 3.6%, 2.7%, and 2.0%, respectively. All precision results on the c502 module were within the stated limits except for fructosamine and transferrin. Neither assay met the minimum precision requirements of 2.6% and 2.3%. Estradiol was the only assay on the e602 module outside the desirable precision limits for the serum control, but within the minimum precision limit of 17.1%.

Results of Trueness Evaluations

Estimates of uncertainty used to assess trueness provided by Roche Diagnostics (Indianapolis, IN) are shown in columns 6 and 7 of **Table 2**. Uncertainty results that exceeded the desirable bias limits were highlighted in red. On the ISE module, chloride and sodium just exceeded the desirable bias limits of 0.5% and 0.3% with uncertainty limits of 0.7% and 0.5%. Using the minimum bias limit defined as <0.350 $(CV_I^2 + CV_A^2)^{\frac{1}{2}}$,[15] both levels of reference material for chloride and level 1 of sodium were within the minimum bias limit of 0.7% and 0.4%, respectively, but level 2 of sodium was still outside even the minimum bias limit. All assays were within the desirable bias limits on the c701 except for calcium and magnesium. Calcium was just outside the desirable uncertainty limit of 0.8%, with an uncertainty of 0.9%, but was within the minimum bias limit of 1.2%. Magnesium was also within the minimum bias limit of 2.7% with an uncertainty of 2.3%. All assays were within the desirable bias limits on the c502 and the e602.

Results of Linearity Assessments

Ranges of smallest and largest observed slopes from least squared linear regression analysis of linearity material or diluted serum pools across multiple cobas 8000 analyzers are shown in column 8 of **Table 2**. Slopes from the linear regression analysis were compared with the CAP performance limits given in **Table 1**. All assays for the

Table 2
Evaluation of Roche cobas 8000 analyzer relative to performance goals for imprecision, trueness, linearity, detection limit, and consistency among instruments and over time

			Precision		Trueness					Consistency	
Mod	Assay	Material	Intra-assay[b] (%CV)	Interassay[a] (%CV)	Level	Uncertainty	Linearity[a]	Detect Limit	Decision Level	Instrument Bias (%)	Time Bias (%)
ISE	Chloride	QC	0.3–0.6	1.0–1.2	1	0.6	0.9973–1.0045	60	100	0.0	0.4
		Serum	0.2–1.3	1.3–1.7	2	0.7	—	—	108	0.1	0.4
ISE	Potassium	QC	0.0–0.5	1.1–1.8	1	0.7	0.9952–0.9992	1.5c	3.6	1.2	0.2
		Serum	0.0–1.6	1.4–2.6	2	0.7	—	—	5.2	0.5	0.5
ISE	Sodium	QC	0.2–0.4	0.6–1.4	1	0.4	0.9918–0.9986	80	134	0.2	1.1
		Serum	0.3–1.2	0.8–1.3	2	0.5	—	—	145	0.0	1.2
c701	Alanine aminotransferase	QC	2.3–3.8	3.9–4.3	1	4.1	1.0002–1.0221	5	7	11.3	2.5
		Serum	1.5–3.0	5.5–7.2	—	—	—	—	45	0.6	3.9
c701	Albumin	QC	1.0–2.1	2.2–2.3	1	1.0	1.0033–1.0067	0.2	3.5	0.9	3.2
		Serum	1.5–1.9	1.6–2.4	—	—	—	—	5	0.9	2.1
c701	Alkaline phosphatase	QC	0.8–1.0	1.9–2.6	1	2.4	1.0015–1.0056	5	98	4.9	0.7
		Serum	0.8–1.5	1.2–2.8	—	—	—	—	251	2.5	2.0
c701	Aspartate aminotransferase	QC	1.9–3.8	3.9–4.5	1	2.0	1.0002–1.0045	5	12	15.3	6.0
		Serum	1.9–3.1	3.0–3.5	—	—	—	—	31	6.1	0.8
c701	Bicarbonate	QC	1.4–3.1	2.6–5.9	N/A	N/A	0.9887–0.9984	2	22	1.6	2.8
		Serum	1.3–3.1	2.9–4.0	—	—	—	—	29	2.2	2.0
c701	Blood urea nitrogen	QC	0.0–2.7	1.7–2.5	1	1.2	0.9985–1.0013	2d	6	2.1	8.2
		Serum	0.0–2.3	1.9–2.8	—	—	—	—	21	1.7	1.2
c701	Calcium	QC	0.6–0.7	1.1–1.5	1	0.9	1.0054–1.0104	0.4	8.9	0.8	0.3
		Serum	1.1–1.6	1.6–2.0	—	—	—	—	10.1	0.9	0.1
c701	Cholesterol	QC	0.8–1.1	1.0–1.9	1	0.6	0.9968–1.0016	3.86	200	0.1	1.9
		Serum	1.2–1.6	1.2–1.8	—	—	—	—	240	0.1	2.1
c701	C-Reactive protein	QC	0.8–1.2	2.3–2.8	1	2.1	0.9809–1.0075	3.0d	8	0.2e	3.4e
		Serum	1.7–2.8	1.7–2.8	—	—	—	—	—	—	—
c701	Creatinine	QC	1.1–1.5	1.6–2.1	1	1.4	0.9792–1.0013	0.1d	0.8	3.9	1.6
		Serum	1.1–1.6	1.3–1.8	—	—	—	—	1.3	2.3	2.7
c701	Direct bilirubin	QC	0.0–7.6	10.6–18.5	1	1.2	0.9702–0.9862	0.1c	0.3	2.5	1.3
		Serum	0.0–14.8	10.6–12.9	—	—	—	—	—	—	—

(continued on next page)

Table 2
(continued)

Mod	Assay	Material	Precision Intra-assay[b] (%CV)	Interassay[a] (%CV)	Trueness Level	Uncertainty	Linearity[a]	Detect Limit	Decision Level	Consistency Instrument Bias (%)	Time Bias (%)
c701	Glucose	QC	0.6–1.0	1.4–1.5	1	1.4	0.9911–1.0014	2	70	0.4	0.0
		Serum	0.9–1.7	1.1–1.2	—	—	—	—	100	0.6	0.1
c701	High-density lipoprotein	QC	0.0–1.8	2.1–2.9	1	2.0	0.9942–1.0107	3[c]	40	1.2	0.9
		Serum	1.1–1.5	1.6–2.4	—	—	—	—	60	0.7	1.8
c701	Lactate dehydrogenase	QC	0.5–1.0	1.3–1.9	1	1.5	0.9985–1.0008	10	122	1.5[e]	1.0[e]
		Serum	0.8–1.5	1.5–2.2	—	—	—	—	222	1.4[e]	0.4[e]
c701	Magnesium	QC	0.8–2.0	1.9–2.9	1	2.3	0.9959–1.0023	0.12	1.7	1.4	0.8
		Serum	0.0–1.8	1.5–2.8	—	—	—	—	2.3	1.0	1.3
c701	Phosphorus	QC	0.9–1.7	1.8–2.2	1	2.3	0.9968–1.0025	0.31	2.5	1.5	2.5
		Serum	1.2–2.3	1.5–2.1	—	—	—	—	4.5	0.8	1.1
c701	Total bilirubin	QC	0.0–5.3	4.5–5.0	1	2.1	0.9743–0.9972	0.1[c]	1	1.4	0.4
		Serum	0.0–5.7	7.0–9.1	—	—	—	—	16	1.3	4.6
c701	Total protein	QC	0.7–1.1	1.7–2.1	1	1.2	1.0000–1.0091	0.2	6.3	2.0	2.6
		Serum	1.3–1.6	1.5–2.4	—	—	—	—	7.9	2.0	2.2
c701	Triglycerides	QC	0.9–1.1	1.3–2.0	1	1.1	0.9890–1.0015	8.85	150	1.1	4.4
		Serum	0.9–1.4	1.7–2.4	—	—	—	—	400	0.1	1.0
c701	Uric acid	QC	0.5–1.2	1.0–1.5	1	0.4	0.9966–1.0041	0.2	3.7	1.1	1.5
		Serum	1.2–1.6	1.8–2.4	—	—	—	—	8.0	1.2	0.1
c502	Amylase	QC	0.8–0.9	1.1–1.7	1	0.9	0.9966–1.0100	3	26	5.9	2.8
		Serum	0.5–0.9	0.9–1.7	—	—	—	—	102	1.5	0.3
c502	β-Hydroxybutyrate	QC	0.0–0.0	0.0–11.5	N/A	N/A	0.9920–0.9930	0.1[d]	0.2	2.4	8.7
		Serum	0.0–20.2	16.2–16.2	—	—	—	—	1.0	1.0	737.0
c502	Creatine kinase	QC	0.7–0.8	1.2–1.4	1	1.5	0.9892–1.0027	7	38	0.9[e]	13.7[e]
		Serum	0.7–1.1	2.4–2.5	—	—	—	—	336	1.5[e]	3.8[e]
c502	Fructosamine	QC	1.7–2.8	1.8–2.7	N/A	N/A	0.9973–0.9983	14	200	0.1	1.4
		Serum	1.2–3.2	1.4–3.4	—	—	—	—	285	0.0	0.3
c502	γ-Glutamyltransferase	QC	1.2–1.2	2.1–2.1	1	2.2	0.9955–0.9983	3	7	0.3[e]	15.9[e]
		Serum	0.7–0.9	1.1–1.4	—	—	—	—	48	1.9[e]	2.2[e]

c502	Iron	QC	0.9-1.0	1.3-1.7	1	1.2	1.0003-1.0013	5	3	21.4e	1.9e
		Serum	0.7-0.9	1.6-1.7	—	—	—	—	150	1.5e	1.8e
c502	Lipase	QC	0.0-1.2	2.5-2.8	N/A	N/A	1.0029-1.0055	2	10	3.3e	23.2e
		Serum	0.0-1.0	3.4-5.0	—	—	—	—	73	0.3e	3.5e
c502	Soluble transferrin receptor	QC	2.4-2.6	3.4-3.9	1	5.9	0.98536-0.9858	0.5	1.8	5.3	3.8
		Serum	1.1-2.7	2.2-3.1	5	0.5	—	—	4.6	1.3	3.5
c502	Transferrin	QC	1.4-1.7	1.3-1.6	1	0.9	1.0080-1.0447	10	200	0.1	0.2
		Serum	1.2-2.5	1.2-1.7	—	—	—	—	360	0.6	1.1
e602	C peptide	QC	0.6-1.9	3.4-5.3	1	2.0	1.0121-1.0545	0.1d	1.1	5.8	1.0
		Serum	1.6-2.4	2.0-4.4	2	2.3	—	—	4.4	2.6	0.3
e602	Creatine kinase MB	QC	0.9-1.5	1.4-3.2	1	5.6	0.9551-0.9993	1.0d	3.8	10.8e	2.1e
		Serum	1.1-2.1	2.1-3.3	2	4.6	—	—	6.7	7.2e	0.4e
e602	Digoxin	QC	3.1-6.6	6.5-7.7	2	5.7	0.9046-0.9687	0.3d	0.5	10.3	7.0
		Serum	7.6-19.5	10.9-22.3	2	2.4	—	—	4	6.6	1.2
e602	Estradiol	QC	1.6-3.8	1.6-6.6	1	7.3	0.9112-0.9705	10.0d	15	12.5e	0.6e
		Serum	1.5-3.3	2.9-12.8	2	2.0	—	—	350	2.1e	1.6e
e602	Free prostate-specific antigen	QC	0.8-1.6	1.6-3.0	1	5.6	0.9458-1.0147	0.10d	N/A	N/A	N/A
		Serum	1.8-6.3	2.2-4.2	2	1.2	—	—	N/A	—	—
e602	Human chorionic gonadotropin	QC	1.6-2.4	2.8-4.5	1	7.9	0.9917-1.0427	0.5d	5	2.4e	2.1e
		Serum	1.7-2.2	1.8-3.8	2	1.4	—	—	25	5.4e	1.3e
e602	Insulin	QC	1.1-1.8	2.2-3.3	1	3.9	1.0362-1.0521	0.5d	2.6	8.6e	10.9e
		Serum	1.7-2.5	1.7-2.7	2	1.5	—	—	24.9	0.7e	2.5e
e602	N-Terminal pro b-type natriuretic peptide	QC	1.3-1.8	2.7-4.9	1	1.4	1.0186-1.0635	25d	51	4.0e	1.8e
		Serum	1.9-2.6	2.3-4.1	2	1.4	—	—	500	1.3e	0.3e
e602	Parathyroid hormone	QC	0.8-1.4	2.2-4.7	1	5.5	0.9270-1.0296	6.0d	15	7.7e	5.4e
		Serum	1.4-2.6	4.1-5.9	2	1.8	—	—	65	3.5e	1.5e
e602	Progesterone	QC	2.0-5.0	4.5-9.2	1	43.3	0.9341-0.9665	0.15d	1.5	9.6	9.6
		Serum	2.6-3.2	3.8-6.9	2	3.9	—	—	27	1.4	2.5
e602	Prolactin	QC	1.0-1.4	2.3-4.2	1	53.3	1.0129-1.0529	1.0d	4	13.3	5.7
		Serum	1.5-3.3	2.6-5.5	2	1.8	—	—	23.3	0.1	0.0
e602	Prostate-specific antigen	QC	0.6-1.0	1.6-2.6	—	—	0.9553-1.0333	0.10d	0.3	16.0e	4.4e
		Serum	0.9-2.4	1.5-2.7	2	2.3	—	—	6.1	0.1e	2.3e

(continued on next page)

Table 2
(continued)

Mod	Assay	Material	Precision		Trueness			Detect Limit	Decision Level	Consistency	
			Intra-assay[b] (%CV)	Interassay[a] (%CV)	Level	Uncertainty	Linearity[a]			Instrument Bias (%)	Time Bias (%)
e602	Thyroid-stimulating hormone	QC	0.5–1.0	1.5–3.1	1	1.2	0.9697–1.0493	0.01[d]	0.3	24.6[e]	22.6[e]
		Serum	1.2–2.6	1.8–3.7	—	—	—	—	10	0.8[e]	0.7[e]
e602	Troponin T	QC	1.4–2.3	3.2–5.9	1	1.3	0.9636–1.0047	0.010[d]	0.3	6.3[e]	0.2[e]
		Serum	1.1–13.4	2.2–5.1	2	1.9	—	—	2.0	0.4[e]	5.1[e]

Assays are listed in alphabetical order according to Roche cobas 8000 module.
[a] Smallest and largest observed slope for linearity across multiple modules.
[b] Lowest and highest observed %CV for intra-assay and interassay precision across multiple modules.
[c] Manufacturer's detection limits confirmed by local testing.
[d] Locally determined detection limits.
[e] Based on regression of data points near decision limits.

ISE, c701, and c502 modules were within acceptable limits but digoxin, estradiol, progesterone, and prostate-specific antigen assays showed linear under-recovery, whereas the N-terminal pro b-type natriuretic peptide assay showed linear over-recovery on the e602 module. These assays are highlighted in red on **Table 2**. Estradiol, N-terminal pro b-type natriuretic peptide, and prostrate-specific antigen slope results were within 50% of the recommended total error limits listed on the Westgard.com Web site based on the work of Ricos and colleagues.[16] Total error limits were not available to evaluate the linearity results for digoxin and progesterone.

Results of Assessment of Detection Limits

The detection limits stated by the reagent manufacturer and the detection limits determined locally are shown in column 9 of **Table 2**. The detection limit is marked with a superscript C if the manufacturer's detection limit was confirmed locally. Detection limits determined locally are marked with a superscript D. The manufacturer's claimed detection limit was confirmed or a detection limit was determined locally if the coefficient of variation was less than 10% for troponin T and less than 20% for all other assays. The detection limits shown in **Table 2** were highlighted in gray if they could not be evaluated using the 0.10 percentile established limits. N-terminal pro b-type natriuretic peptide exceeded the 0.10 percentile limits.

Results of Consistency Assessments

The analytical bias between multiple instruments used simultaneously and the analytical bias across time at 2 decision levels are shown in columns 11 and 12 of **Table 2**. Bias limits marked with a superscript B are based on regression analysis of data near the decision limits. Assays were highlighted in red if the observed analytical bias was greater than the clinical performance limits for bias established using the cumulative distribution of patient test values. All assays were within the performance limits on the ISE module except for sodium analytical bias across time at the higher decision level. Sodium was also outside Ricos and colleagues'[16] desirable and minimum bias limits of 0.3% and 0.4%. Alkaline phosphatase, aspartate aminotransferase, and total protein instrument bias exceeded the proposed performance limits at 1 or more decision levels on the c701. Albumin and total protein exceed the performance limits for time bias on the c701. Alkaline phosphatase instrument bias was within the desirable analytical bias limit of 6.4%. Calcium instrument bias was within the minimum bias limit of 1.3%. Aspartate aminotransferase, albumin, and total protein were outside both the desirable and minimum bias performance limits. On the c502, the observed iron instrument bias and creatine kinase, γ-glutamyltransferase, and lipase time bias exceeded the population bias performance limits and both the desirable and minimum bias limits. Creatine kinase MB, estradiol, human chorionic gonadotropin, and thyroid-stimulating hormone instrument bias and N-terminal pro b-type natriuretic peptide time bias exceeded the performance limits on the e602. Creatine kinase MB instrument bias was within the minimum bias limit of 11.7% and insulin time bias was within the desirable bias limit of 15.5%. There was no bias limit defined for digoxin because this analyte is not found in healthy subjects.

DISCUSSION

In the absence of well-defined clinical performance limits for the intended use of these clinical chemistry tests, this article provides recommendations for 5 test characteristics based on published studies of biological variations and patient data collected from patients seen at Mayo Clinic, Rochester. These performance limits were used to evaluate the Roche cobas 8000 measurement system. In general, these chemistry tests performed well, although there were some deficiencies. Our findings are similar to the results reported by the group from Croatia for the Roche 6000.[22] They found inadequate precision for total protein, albumin, calcium, sodium, chloride, and high-density lipoprotein cholesterol. They also found issues with inaccuracy for total protein, calcium, sodium, and chloride.

A group at Laboratory Corporation of America evaluated a smaller Roche instrument, the cobas c111. They found slightly better precision and only sodium had imprecision greater than our recommended goal.[23]

A group from Italy evaluated the Beckman Coulter AU680 analyzer using quality specifications based on biological variation.[24] All analytes, except sodium at 119 mmol/L, met either the desirable or optimum precision goals.

Our study used the traceability values provided by Roche to evaluate trueness and all analytes passed. Investigators in Milano, Italy, measured the accuracy of the serum albumin test on the Roche cobas 501 platform and found it to be much higher, with a combined uncertainty of 6.69% across 2 lots of assay reagents.[25] These estimates included both the uncertainty of the traceability chain and the uncertainty caused by the random effects of measurement. Our trueness parameter relates only to the traceability to reference standards based on large series of measurements performed by the manufacturer.

This article provides recommendations for 5 analytical performance goals that are specific for many general chemistry analytes. Although these goals are not based on well-controlled clinical outcome studies, they do relate to clinical practice and therefore serve as surrogate clinical goals. The Roche 8000 analytical system meets many, but not all, of these requirements. Many instruments have similar performance characteristics and therefore would meet many, but not all, of these performance goals.

As medical laboratories implement new guidelines for risk management, it is still critical to show that safety characteristics are acceptable for the intended clinical use of laboratory tests. Quality control plans may implement many different controls to monitor the performance of an analytical system, but those controls primarily measure changes in performance and do not verify that performance is acceptable for the intended use. Risk management must be implemented with an understanding of the critical steps required for analytical quality management.

REFERENCES

1. Middle JG, Kane JW. Oestradiol assays: fitness for purpose? Ann Clin Biochem 2009;46:441–56.
2. Thompson M, Ellison SL, Wood R. Harmonized guidelines for single laboratory validation of methods of analysis (IUPAC technical report). Pure Appl Chem 2002;74(5):835–55.
3. Tate J, Panteghini M. Standardisation - the theory and the practice. Clin Biochem Rev 2007;28:127–30.
4. BIVDA. Directive 98/79/EC of the European Parliament and of the Council of 27 October 1998 on in vitro diagnostic medical devices. Official Journal of the European Communities 1998;41:L331/331-L331/337.
5. BIVDA. Revision of Directive 98/79/EC of the European Parliament and of the Council of 27 October 1998 on in vitro diagnostic medical devices. Public consultation. European Commission, Health and Consumers Directorate-General. Official Journal of the European Communities 2010(June 2010).

6. BIVDA. Revision of Directive 98/79/EC of the European Parliament and of the Council of 27 October 1998 on in vitro diagnostic medical devices. Summary responses to the Public Consultation. European Commission, Health and Consumers Directorate-General. Official Journal of the European Communities 2011.
7. Jhang JS, Chang CC, Fink DJ, et al. Evaluation of linearity in the clinical laboratory. Arch Pathol Lab Med 2004;128(1):44–8.
8. Tholen DW, Kroll M, Astles JR, et al, editors. Evaluation of the linearity of quantitative measurement procedures: a statistical approach; approved guideline, EP06-A, vol. 23. Clinical and Laboratory Standards Institute; 2003.
9. CAP. 2012 Calibration verification/linearity program user's guide. Northfield: College of American Pathologist; 2012.
10. Westgard JO. The meaning and application of total error. [World Wide Web]. 2007. Available at: http://www.westgard/essay111.htm. Accessed October 5, 2012.
11. Kroll MH, Praestgaard J, Michaliszyn E, et al. Evaluation of the extent of nonlinearity in reportable range studies. Arch Pathol Lab Med 2000;124(9):1331–8.
12. Kroll MH, Emancipator K. A theoretical evaluation of linearity. Clin Chem 1993; 39(3):405–13.
13. Emancipator K, Kroll M. A quantitative measure of nonlinearity. Clin Chem 1993; 39(5):766–72.
14. Young D, Friedman R. 4th edition. Effects of disease on clinical laboratory tests, vols. 1 and 2. Washington, DC: AACC Press; 2001.
15. Fraser CG, Petersen PH. Analytical performance characteristics should be judged against objective quality specifications. Clin Chem 1999;45(3):321–3.
16. Ricos C, Alvarez V, Cava F, et al. Current databases on biologic variation: pros, cons and progress. Scand J Clin Lab Invest 1999;59(7):491–500.
17. Westgard JO. Desirable specifications for total error, imprecision, and bias, derived from intra- and inter-individual biologic variation. 2012. Available at: www.westgard.com/biodatabase1.htm. Accessed October 5, 2012.
18. Klee G, Schryver P, Kisabeth R. Analytic bias specifications based on the analysis of effects on performance of medical guidelines. Scand J Clin Lab Invest 1999;59(7):509–12.
19. Klee GG. A conceptual model for establishing tolerance limits for analytic bias and imprecision based on variations in population test distributions. Clin Chim Acta 1997;260(2):175–88.
20. Klee GG. Establishment of outcome-related analytic performance goals. Clin Chem 2010;56(5):714–22.
21. BIPM, editor. The guide to the expression of uncertainty in measurement. 1st edn. Geneve, Switzerland: International Organization for Standardization; 1993.
22. Smolcic V, Bilic-Zulle L, Fisic E. Validation of methods performance for routine biochemistry analytes at cobas 6000 analyzer series module C501. Biochem Med 2011;21(2):182–90.
23. Bowling J, Katayev A. An evaluation of the Roche cobas C111. Lab Med 2010; 41(7):398–402.
24. Cattozzo G, Albeni C, Calonaci A, et al. Evaluation of the analytical performance of the Beckman Coulter AU680 automated analytical system based on quality specifications for allowable performance derived from biological variation. Clin Chem Lab Med 2011;49(9):1563–7.
25. Ilenia I, Braga F, Mozzi R, et al. Is the accuracy of serum albumin measurements suitable for clinical application of the test? Clin Chim Acta 2011;412(9–10):791–2.

Validating the Performance of QC Procedures

John Yundt-Pacheco, MSCS, Curtis A. Parvin, PhD*

KEYWORDS

- Quality control • Out-of-control condition • QC performance evaluation
- Statistical QC

KEY POINTS

- The performance of quality control procedures can be validated by assessing the expected number of unreliable patient results produced because of an out-of-control condition for a given quality control strategy and determining if the risk of producing and reporting unreliable patient results is acceptable.
- The expected number of unreliable patient results reported before and after the last accepted quality control evaluation before the detection of an out-of-control condition can be used as design criteria for quality control strategies that meet a laboratory's risk criteria.
- A methodology for computing the expected number of unreliable patient results produced because of an out-of-control condition for a given quality control strategy is presented.

INTRODUCTION TO QC PERFORMANCE VALIDATION

With the introduction of risk management for development of laboratory quality control (QC) plans, many different types of controls may be used to monitor the performance of an analytical process and hopefully detect any errors that may occur. Some of these controls are provided by the manufacturer and built into the analyzer. Others, such as statistical QC procedures, are implemented by the laboratory to provide an independent monitor of performance. Still others are implemented by the laboratory to monitor specific faults or causes of errors, such as specimen integrity and suitability for analysis. Given that the purpose of the QC plan is to detect problems that may occur, it is important to evaluate the detection capabilities of different controls and ensure they will indeed be able to detect medically important errors.

For some controls (eg, training of analysts), it is difficult to assess their effectiveness. For other controls, such as those implemented by the manufacturer (eg, short sample detector), the manufacturer should have experimental evidence to prove the

Quality Systems Division, Bio-Rad Laboratories, 3201 Technology Drive, Plano, TX 75074, USA
* Corresponding author.
E-mail address: Curtis_Parvin@Bio-Rad.com

effectiveness of the control. Unfortunately, manufacturers are not required to disclose their studies and the laboratory is unlikely to be able to perform studies to prove the effectiveness of a manufacturer's controls. Such studies require the introduction of faults (eg, shorted samples by 10%, 20%, 30%, and so forth), to experimentally verify the detection characteristic of the short sample control.

Fortunately, laboratories can validate the effectiveness of statistical QC (SQC) procedures. SQC procedures provide an independent control that the laboratory can design and verify that the performance characteristics are appropriate for the intended use of laboratory tests. The focus of this discussion, therefore, is on how a laboratory can validate the performance of SQC procedures.

Validate That You Have a Reasonable QC Strategy

The validation of a QC procedure can be thought of as answering the question "Does my QC procedure meet my expectations?" Unfortunately, this quickly leads to the question "What are my expectations with respect to my QC procedure performance?" This question is usually answered with some form of "My QC procedure should catch clinically significant errors." Traditionally, the validation of a QC procedure has focused on assessing whether it has sufficient power (a high enough probability) to detect any "critical" out-of-control conditions that would compromise an unacceptably high fraction of patient examinations (say, 5% or more) in the presence of the out-of-control condition.[1–3]

The traditional approach to QC validation was formulated in an era of batch testing in which there was a direct correlation between the quality of a control material examination and the patient specimen examinations in the batch. With discrete testing, where each specimen is examined individually, there is no longer the direct correlation between the quality of a control specimen and the quality of a subsequent patient specimen. Even if a QC procedure could guarantee that the test system was not in an out-of-control state at the time the QC evaluation was performed, it cannot ensure the quality of subsequent patient specimen examinations because an out-of-control condition could occur after the QC evaluation that would adversely affect the patient specimens evaluated until the next QC evaluation is performed.

Define Performance Metric

In the age of risk management, a different performance metric is required to judge the efficacy of QC strategies whether they are deployed on batch-testing systems or discrete testing systems. As the focus of risk management is the patient, so too should the focus of QC procedure validation be the patient. Specifically, the question becomes "How are patient specimen examinations affected by an out-of-control condition that occurs while a particular QC strategy is used?" This question can be reframed as "For a given QC strategy, what is the expected number of unreliable patient specimen results produced when an out-of-control condition exists on the evaluation instrument?" As each magnitude of an out-of-control condition may produce a different expected number of unreliable patient specimen results and there is no way of knowing what size of out-of-control condition will occur, the QC validation question becomes "Is the expected number of unreliable patient specimen results produced for any size of an out-of-control condition acceptable?"[4] This article focuses on how to compute for a given QC strategy the expected number of unreliable patient results produced as a result of an out-of-control condition (abbreviated $E[N_u]$) and how to use it to validate the acceptability of a QC strategy.[5] Here, a QC strategy is composed of a QC schedule (how often do QC events occur), the number of QC specimens evaluated at each QC event, and the QC rule(s) applied to the QC specimen results.

What Is Reasonable Performance?

The ability to compute $E(N_u)$ for a given QC strategy is insufficient for validation. The validation question asks "Is the maximum $E(N_u)$ for a given quality control strategy on a given analyte acceptable?" There is no universally correct answer to this. A laboratory's tolerance for maximum $E(N_u)$ on a given analyte should be informed by how the analyte results are used by treating physicians, and what is possible given the resource constraints of the laboratory. A laboratory needs to decide what is appropriate for each analyte and design QC procedures accordingly.[6]

The first step in validating a QC strategy is to specify the quality required in a patient result. This answers the question "How much error makes a result unreliable?"

QUALITY SPECIFICATIONS
What Is an Unreliable Result?

The first step in designing (and validating) QC procedures is to determine how much error in a specimen result is unacceptable. There has been a great deal of thought and effort put into determining how to best assign a quality specification that can be used to classify results as acceptable or unacceptable.[7,8] This topic is not addressed here, instead the focus here will be on using a quality specification for validating QC procedures.

Although there are many ways to specify how much quality is needed for a particular analyte, we will use an allowable total error specification (TE_a) expressed as a percentage. TE_a is usually specified as a single value, but in some cases it may be concentration based with different specifications given at different concentrations. The critical issue is to have TE_a specifications that reflect the quality required by those who use the results to diagnose and treat patients.

Unreliable = Incorrect = Unacceptable

When a reported specimen result differs from the correct specimen value by more than TE_a, the result is deemed to be unreliable. Note that it is not easy to know what the correct value of a specimen result is, as the analytical process always has some measure of inherent error. An unreliable result may also be known as an incorrect or an unacceptable result. These are synonyms for results with a difference from the correct analyte concentration that is larger than TE_a. Ideally, the amount of inherent analytical error will be small compared with TE_a when the analytical system is operating normally (in an in-control state). **Fig. 1** plots an example measurement error frequency distribution for an in-control process showing the inherent imprecision of the analytical process relative to the allowable total error specification for the analyte.

Probability of Producing Unreliable Results When the System Is in Control

There is always some probability of producing an unreliable result even when the analysis system is functioning normally in an in-control state. A QC strategy is designed to detect changes from the analytical system's in-control state. The efficacy of a QC strategy should be measured by how many additional unreliable results are produced during an out-of-control condition above the number of unreliable results produced when the system is in control. $E(N_u)$ is the expected number of unreliable patient results produced because of an out-of-control condition for a given QC strategy.

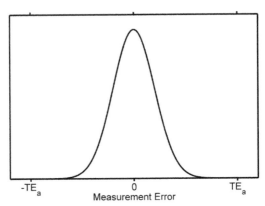

Fig. 1. Example measurement error distribution with specified allowable total error (TE$_a$) limits.

Sigma Metric: A Measure of In-Control Capability

The sigma metric, $sigma = \dfrac{TE_a - |bias|}{CV}$, is computed as the ratio of the allowable total error adjusted for bias, to the stable in-control analytical imprecision. The sigma metric can be used to assess how likely an analytical system is to produce unreliable results during in-control operation.[9]

Sigma metrics are also an easy way to judge how tolerant an analytical process is to out-of-control conditions. For example, if 1,000,000 patient specimens are evaluated on a 6-sigma process in the presence of an out-of-control condition that produces a 2-SD shift in the process, an additional 32 results are expected to be unreliable. On the other hand, if 1,000,000 patient specimens are evaluated on a 2-sigma process with a 2-SD out-of-control shift in the process, an additional 454,531 results are expected to be unreliable (**Fig. 2**).

The lower the sigma metric, the higher the E(N$_u$) will be for a given out-of-control condition. In general, low sigma processes require more QC resources than high sigma processes to produce an equivalent E(N$_u$).

OUT-OF-CONTROL CONDITIONS
Transient versus Persistent Out-of-Control Conditions

Although sigma metrics can provide guidance on how rapidly unreliable results are expected to accumulate in the presence of an out-of-control condition and what kind of a QC strategy is necessary for mitigation, it should be noted that the periodic assessment of QC materials will do little to mitigate transient out-of-control conditions.[10]

Transient out-of-control conditions are system malfunctions that exist for some period of time and then disappear without any overt action taken. They may be caused by something like a power irregularity or a manufacturing defect in some subset of consumables. These types of transient out-of-control conditions are generally beyond the scope of traditional QC measures and are very difficult to identify. By their nature, their impact on the quality of patient specimen results is limited.

Persistent out-of-control conditions are system malfunctions that persist until they are identified and corrected. Persistent out-of-control conditions are the target of QC testing. From a validation standpoint, QC strategies are evaluated by their efficacy at limiting the production of unreliable results in the presence of a persistent

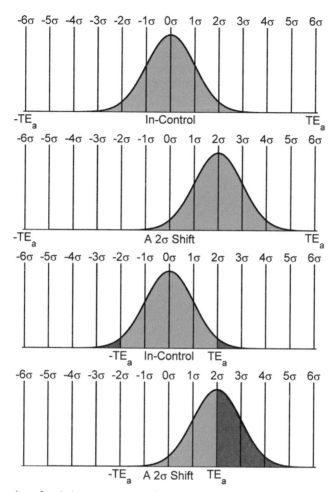

Fig. 2. Examples of a 6-sigma process and a 2-sigma process. The upper 2 figures show measurement error distributions for an in-control process (*top*) and an out-of-control process with a 2-SD (2σ) shift (*second from top*) and an allowable total error (TE$_a$) specification of ±6σ. The bottom 2 figures show measurement error distributions for an in-control process (*second from bottom*) and an out-of-control process with a 2-SD (2σ) shift (*bottom*) and an allowable total error (TE$_a$) specification of ±2σ. The areas shaded in green represent the likelihood of producing results that meet the specified quality requirement. The areas shaded in red represent the likelihood of producing results that fail to meet the specified quality requirement.

out-of-control condition. For the purpose of validation, it is assumed that an out-of-control condition will be rectified only when a QC evaluation is rejected (ie, the malfunction is identified as a result of a failed QC evaluation).[11]

The expected number of unreliable patient specimen results produced because of an out-of-control condition can be computed as the product of the average number of patients examined while the out-of-control condition exists and the probability of the analytical system producing unreliable results in the presence of the out-of-control condition.[12,13]

The Difference in the Probability of Producing Unreliable Results During an Out-of-Control Condition: The ΔP_E Curve

It should be intuitive that a large out-of-control condition will have a high probability of producing unreliable results and that a very small out-of-control condition will have almost no effect on the probability of producing unreliable results. The probability of producing unreliable results can be computed when the analytical system is operating in its in-control state. The probability will depend on the allowable total error specification and the analytical system's imprecision and bias. The probability may depend on specimen concentration. For a given magnitude of out-of-control condition, the probability of producing unreliable results can also be computed. The difference in the probabilities of producing unreliable results in the out-of-control state and the in-control state is denoted ΔP_E. If ΔP_E varies with specimen concentration, then averaging ΔP_E over the frequency distribution of patient specimen concentrations will give a representative ΔP_E for the analytical process.

When a process is in its in-control state, $\Delta P_E = 0$. For a large enough out-of-control condition, ΔP_E will approach 1. Computing ΔP_E for out-of-control conditions that range in magnitude from 0 (in control) to 2 times the allowable total error specification ($2TE_a$) will produce a ΔP_E curve that transitions from 0 to near 1 as a function of the magnitude of the out-of-control condition. **Fig. 3** gives an example of such a ΔP_E curve. In this figure, SE denotes a systematic-error out-of-control condition that causes a shift in the measurement process. The magnitude of the shift is expressed in multiples of the in-control analytical imprecision of the process.

DETECTING AN OUT-OF-CONTROL CONDITION

The expected number of unreliable patient results produced because of an out-of-control condition is the product of ΔP_E and the average number of patient specimens evaluated during the existence of the out-of-control condition. It is assumed that the out-of-control condition will persist until it is identified by a QC rejection. The average number of patient specimens evaluated while the out-of-control condition persists will depend on the power of the QC rule(s) used and the number of patient specimens evaluated between QC events.

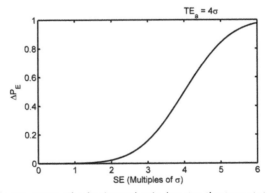

Fig. 3. An example ΔP_E curve. The horizontal axis denotes the true state of the analytical process. SE represents a systematic error out-of-control condition in multiples of the stable analytical imprecision of the process (σ). A value of SE = 0 implies the analytical process is in an in-control state. ΔP_E denotes the change in the probability of producing patient results that fail to meet the specified allowable total error specification (TE_a) as a function of the magnitude of the out-of-control state.

In general, large out-of-control conditions are easy to detect and small out-of-control conditions are difficult to detect. For a very large out-of-control condition, just about any QC rule will detect it at the first QC event after it occurs, but for a small out-of-control condition, it may require several QC events after it occurs before the QC rule(s) will detect it.

QC Rules Have Different Error Detection Power

The probability that a QC rule will reject, given an out-of-control condition of a certain size, is called the QC rule's error detection power. The probability of error detection is denoted P_{ed}. This probability can be computed across a range from no out-of-control condition (in-control state) to very large out-of-control conditions to form a power curve (**Fig. 4**). Different QC rules will have different power curves. The power curves for a variety of QC rules have been well documented.[14–16] Repeating a QC rule on a second set of QC specimen evaluations as part of a QC strategy will have a different P_{ed} than using the QC rule on a single sample.[17]

HOW LONG HAS THE ERROR BEEN PRESENT?

The expected (or average) number of QC events required to detect an out-of-control condition of a given magnitude is related to the probability of a QC rule rejection represented by the power curve. There is an inverse relationship between the probability of a QC rule rejection and the average number of QC events required to detect the out-of-control condition; the higher the probability of error detection, the lower the average number of QC events required to detect the out-of-control condition. For QC rules that evaluate only the control specimen results produced in the current QC event, the average number of QC events to detection is $1/P_{ed}$. For example, in the power curve depicted in **Fig. 4**, there is about a 40% chance of a QC rule rejection for an out-of-control condition equivalent to a 2-SD shift. Therefore, on average, it will take 2.5 QC events to detect a 2-SD out-of-control shift in the analytical test system. For QC rules that incorporate control specimen results from more than a single QC event, an inverse relationship between the probability of a QC rule rejection and the average

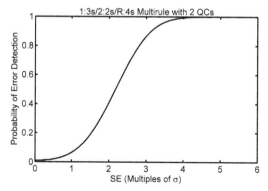

Fig. 4. An example power curve for a 1:3s/2:2s/R:4s QC multirule[14] testing 2 concentration levels of QC. The horizontal axis denotes the true state of the analytical process. SE represents a systematic error out-of-control condition in multiples of the stable analytical imprecision of the process (σ). A value of SE = 0 implies the analytical process is in an in-control state. The vertical axis denotes the probability of a QC rule rejection as a function of the magnitude of the out-of-control state.

number of QC events required to detect the out-of-control condition still exists, but it is more complicated.[18]

For any given QC rule and magnitude of out-of-control condition, the expected number of QC events needed to detect the out-of-control condition can be computed. Combining the expected number of QC events needed to detect the out-of-control condition with the average number of patient specimens examined between QC events gives a measure of how many patient specimens are predicted to be affected by a persistent out-of-control condition before it is identified and resolved (**Fig. 5**).[19]

The expected number of patients affected curve depicts how many patient specimens will be evaluated between the occurrence of an out-of-control condition of a given magnitude and a QC rule rejection. When the analysis system is in control (SE = 0), the expected number is large, reflecting the number of patient specimens evaluated between QC rule false rejections. A QC rule false rejection is a QC rule rejection that occurs when there is no out-of-control condition present. In the example depicted in **Fig. 5**, an average of 100 patient specimens are examined between QC events and the QC rule's false rejection rate is approximately 0.01. Therefore, we would expect a QC rule false rejection to occur on average about every 1/0.01 = 100 QC events. With an average of 100 patient specimens between QC events, the expected number of patient specimen results between QC rule rejections for the in-control system is 100*100 = 10,000.

The larger the magnitude of the out-of-control condition, the greater the likelihood of a QC rule rejection and the fewer number of QC events needed for detection leading to a lower expected number of patient specimens affected. For a large enough out-of-control condition, a QC rule rejection will be ensured the first time the QC rule is evaluated after the out-of-control condition occurs. Assuming that out-of-control conditions can occur with equal likelihood at any point in the testing process, then the expected number of affected patient results will be one-half the average number of patient specimens evaluated between QC events in the presence of an extremely large out-of-control condition that is detected at the first QC event after its occurrence.

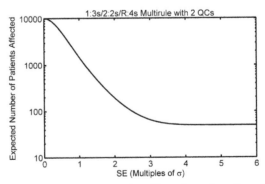

Fig. 5. The expected number of patient results affected as a function of the magnitude of the out-of-control state for a 1:3s/2:2s/R:4s QC multirule[14] testing 2 concentration levels of QC. The horizontal axis denotes the true state of the analytical process. SE represents a systematic error out-of-control condition in multiples of the stable analytical imprecision of the process (σ). A value of SE = 0 implies the analytical process is in an in-control state. The vertical axis denotes the expected number of patient results affected by the out-of-control condition plotted on a log scale.

Frequency of QC Events

The expected number of patient specimen results affected by an out-of-control condition is directly proportional to the average number of patient specimens examined between QC events and therefore is inversely related to the frequency of QC testing. If the frequency of QC testing is doubled (the average number of patient specimens between QC events is halved) then the expected number of patient specimen results affected will be halved. If the frequency of QC testing is halved (the average number of patient specimens between QC events is doubled) then the expected number of patient specimen results affected will be doubled.

EXPECTED NUMBER OF UNRELIABLE PATIENT RESULTS PRODUCED BECAUSE OF AN OUT-OF-CONTROL CONDITION

The expected number of unreliable patient results produced because of an out-of-control condition can be computed as the product of the ΔP_E curve and the expected number of patients affected curve (denoted ANP$_{affected}$ in **Fig. 6**).[12,13] E(N$_u$) increases as the size of the out-of-control condition increases until it reaches a maximum at one-half the average number of patient specimens between QC events.

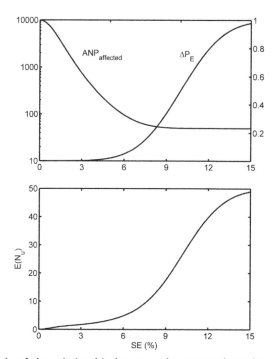

Fig. 6. An example of the relationship between the expected number of patient results affected by an out-of-control condition (ANP$_{affected}$), the difference in the probability of producing unreliable patient results because of the out-of-control condition (ΔP_E), and the expected number of unreliable results produced because of the out-of-control condition (E[N$_u$]). SE represents the magnitude of the systematic error out-of-control condition given as a percentage. E(N$_u$) is the product of ANP$_{affected}$ and ΔP_E.

$E(N_u)$ Is One-Half the Number of Patients Between QCs for Large Errors

If patient specimen results are immediately reported when they are available, they will always be vulnerable to an out-of-control condition that occurs after the last acceptable QC event. Consider an out-of-control condition large enough to make the results from all patient specimens tested while it is present unreliable, and also large enough so that it will be detected by the first QC event while it is present. In the worst case, the out-of-control condition starts between the last accepted QC event and the first patient specimen so that results for all patient specimens evaluated before the next QC event will be unreliable. In the best case, the out-of-control condition starts right after the last patient specimen, but before the next QC event, so that it is detected and resolved before any patient specimens are affected. Under the assumption that an out-of-control condition is equally likely to occur anywhere, the probability that the out-of-control event occurred right after the last accepted QC event is equal to the probability that the out-of-control event occurred right after the last patient specimen before the next QC event. On average the out-of-control event occurs in the middle, so that one-half the number of patient specimen results between QCs will be unreliable. The general rule of thumb for estimating the impact of a large out-of-control condition is that one-half the number of patient specimens between QC events will have unreliable results.[20]

An $E(N_u)$ Cartoon

It is helpful to have a depiction of the analytical process under an out-of-control condition to analyze the relationships between QC rules, QC frequency, and the production of unreliable results (**Fig. 7**).

In the depiction, the horizontal line represents the analytical process over time. The up-shifted line represents the occurrence of an out-of-control condition. The vertical lines represent patient specimens being examined. The diamonds represent QC events; indicated in green for an accepted QC event and red for a rejected QC event. The red asterisks represent unreliable patient specimen results. $E(N_u)$ represents the expected number of red asterisks given the magnitude of the out-of-control condition, the frequency of QC events, and the power of the QC rule.[12]

In the $E(N_u)$ depiction, an out-of-control condition starts after the second QC event. It has a moderate probability of producing unreliable results and 3 are produced before the third QC event that fails to detect the out-of-control condition. It is only at the fifth QC event (the third QC event after the onset of the out-of-control condition) that the out-of-control condition is detected and remedied. An acceptable QC event restarts patient specimen testing and the analytical process continues. Note that not all the patient specimens evaluated during the out-of-control condition had unreliable results (the probability of producing an unreliable results was not 1), and that it took 3 tries to detect the out-of-control condition (the P_{ed} of the QC rule to detect this magnitude of out-of-control condition was presumably approximately one-third).

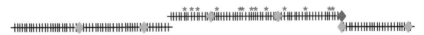

Fig. 7. A depiction of the expected number of unreliable results (represented by the *asterisks*) produced because of an out-of-control condition (the *up-shifted line*). Each vertical line represents a patient specimen examination. Each diamond represents a QC event; a green diamond signifies QC acceptance and a red diamond signifies QC rejection.

Dividing $E(N_u)$ into $E(N_{uf})$ and $E(N_{uc})$

$E(N_u)$ provides a metric that directly relates the reliability of the patient results produced to the performance of a QC strategy subjected to an out-of-control condition of a given size. $E(N_u)$ can be separated into those unreliable patient results that were produced between the onset of the out-of-control condition and the last accepted QC event, and those unreliable patient results that were evaluated between the last accepted QC event and the QC event that detected the out-of-control condition. The expected number of unreliable results produced before the last accepted QC can be deemed "final" results, as the passage of time makes it unlikely that they will be identified and corrected. They are abbreviated $E(N_{uf})$. The expected number of unreliable results produced after the last accepted QC can be deemed "correctable" results, as they have been most recently produced. They are abbreviated $E(N_{uc})$. In **Fig. 8**, $E(N_{uf}) = 9$ (there are 9 red asterisks from the onset of the out-of-control condition to the last accepted QC) and $E(N_{uc}) = 4$ (there are 4 red asterisks between the last accepted QC and the rejected QC).

Computing $E(N_{uf})$

The expected number of "final" unreliable results can be estimated as the product of the expected number of patient specimens affected between the onset of the out-of-control condition and the last accepted QC event (ANP_{pre}) and the difference in the probability of producing unreliable patient results because of the out-of-control condition (ΔP_E). **Fig. 9** shows an example of an $E(N_{uf})$ curve computed over a range of magnitudes of out-of-control conditions.

Using $E(N_{uf})$ to Validate Final Patient Result Quality

Assuming that results before the last accepted QC event are final, $E(N_{uf})$ estimates how many of them will be unreliable because of an out-of-control condition. The $E(N_{uf})$ curve is low for both very small and very large out-of-control conditions and attains its maximum value somewhere in between. If the maximum $E(N_{uf})$ value is deemed acceptable, then the laboratory can be assured that for any out-of-control condition, their QC strategy will limit the expected number of final unreliable patient results reported to an acceptable level. If the maximum possible $E(N_{uf})$ is not deemed acceptable, then the QC strategy (the QC rule, number of control materials used, and the average number of patient specimens evaluated between QC events) should be scrutinized and adjusted until an acceptable maximum $E(N_{uf})$ is achieved. Other things that may need to be considered when evaluating the acceptability of the maximum $E(N_{uf})$ is the size of the out-of-control condition at which it occurs and the TE_a specification.[12,13]

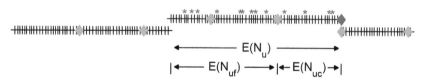

Fig. 8. The total expected number of unreliable results produced because of an out-of-control condition ($E[N_u]$) can be separated into the expected number of unreliable results produced between the inception of the out-of-control condition and the last accepted QC event ($E[N_{uf}]$) and the expected number of unreliable results produced between the last accepted QC event and the QC rule rejection ($E[N_{uc}]$).

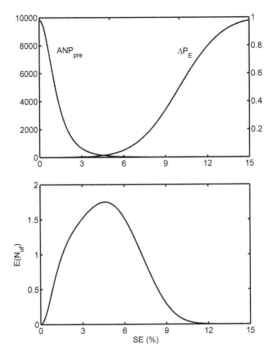

Fig. 9. An example of the relationship between the expected number of patient results affected by an out-of-control condition between its inception and the last accepted QC event (ANP$_{pre}$), the difference in the probability of producing unreliable patient results because of the out-of-control condition (ΔP_E), and the expected number of unreliable results produced between the inception of the out-of-control condition and the last accepted QC event (E[N$_{uf}$]). SE represents the magnitude of the systematic error out-of-control condition given as a percentage. E(N$_{uf}$) is the product of ANP$_{pre}$ and ΔP_E.

Computing E(N$_{uc}$)

The expected number of "correctable" unreliable patient results can be estimated as the product of the expected number of patient specimens affected between the last accepted QC event and the QC event that detected the out-of-control condition (ANP$_{post}$) and the difference in the probability of producing unreliable patient results because of the out-of-control condition (ΔP_E). **Fig. 10** shows an example of an E(N$_{uc}$) curve computed over a range of magnitudes of out-of-control conditions.

The expected number of patient specimens affected between the last accepted QC event and the rejected QC event will depend on whether or not the out-of-control condition is detected at the first QC event after the occurrence of the out-of-control condition. If the out-of-control condition is not detected at the first QC event after it occurs, then all patient specimens between the last accepted QC event and the rejected QC event will have been affected by the out-of-control condition. On the other hand, if the out-of-control condition is detected at the first QC event after it occurs, then as explained earlier, we expect that one-half of the average number of patient specimens examined between QC events would be affected.[19]

The maximum E(N$_{uc}$) value will always be close to one-half the average number of patient specimens examined between QC events. Assuming the laboratory will reevaluate and correct patient specimen results as necessary after an out-of-control condition has been identified and resolved, the maximum E(N$_{uc}$) value should be considered

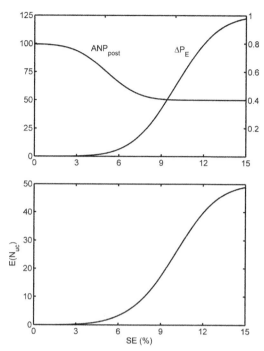

Fig. 10. An example of the relationship between the expected number of patient results affected by an out-of-control condition between the last accepted QC event and the QC rule rejection (ANP_{post}), the difference in the probability of producing unreliable patient results because of the out-of-control condition (ΔP_E), and the expected number of unreliable results produced between the last accepted QC event and the QC rule rejection ($E[N_{uc}]$). SE represents the magnitude of the systematic error out-of-control condition given as a percentage. $E(N_{uc})$ is the product of ANP_{post} and ΔP_E.

the expected number of patient specimens that would need to be corrected in a timely fashion to prevent unreliable patient results being acted on inappropriately if a large out-of-control condition occurs. If a laboratory has procedures in place to be able to identify, repeat, and correct in a timely fashion up to half the average number of patient specimens examined between QC events, then the maximum $E(N_{uc})$ value is acceptable. Otherwise, steps should be taken to reduce the maximum $E(N_{uc})$ value. Reducing the maximum $E(N_{uc})$ value almost always means changing QC frequency.

SUMMARY

A QC strategy consists of the number of control material specimens evaluated during a QC event, the QC rule(s) used to interpret the control results, and how often QC events are scheduled (how many patient specimens are evaluated between QC events). Validating a QC strategy in terms that are directly related to the reporting of reliable patient results can be accomplished by computing the maximum $E(N_{uf})$ and $E(N_{uc})$ values and determining if they are acceptable to the laboratory.

If the maximum $E(N_{uf})$ value is too high, it can be reduced by altering the QC strategy using some combination of increasing the number of control material specimens evaluated during an event, using a QC rule with a higher P_{ed}, or decreasing the number of patient specimens evaluated between QC events. The maximum $E(N_{uf})$ value can also be decreased by reducing the analytical system imprecision or increasing the TE_a specification (neither of which may be an option).

The maximum $E(N_{uc})$ value depends on the average number of patient specimens examined between QC events. If the maximum $E(N_{uc})$ value is too high, lower the number of patient specimens evaluated between QC events.

REFERENCES

1. Westgard JO. How to establish control limits. In: Assuring the right quality right. Madison (WI): Westgard QC, Inc.; 2007. p. 245–59.
2. Brooks ZC. Choosing our own rules. In: Performance-driven quality control. Washington, DC: AACC Press; 2001. p. 89–114.
3. Cembrowski GS, Carey RN. Design of quality control procedures to meet quality specifications. In: Laboratory quality management. Chicago: ASCP Press; 1989. p. 165–85.
4. Parvin CA. Quality-control (QC) performance measures and the QC planning process. Clin Chem 1997;43:602–7.
5. Parvin CA. Statistical topics in the laboratory sciences. In: Ambrosius WT, editor. Topics in biostatistics. Totowa (NJ): Humana Press; 2007. p. 353–75.
6. Cooper G, Dejong N, Ehrmeyer S, et al. Collective opinion paper on findings of the 2010 convocation of experts on laboratory quality. Clin Chem Lab Med 2011;49(5):793–802.
7. Kenny D, Fraser CG, Petersen PH, et al. Consensus agreement. Scand J Clin Lab Invest 1999;59:585.
8. Fraser CG. Quality specifications. In: Biological variation: from principles to practice. Washington, DC: AACC Press; 2001. p. 29–66.
9. Westgard JO. How to use sigma-metrics QC selection tool. In: Assuring the right quality right. Madison (WI): Westgard QC, Inc.; 2007. p. 125–46.
10. Parvin CA. Evaluation of the performance of randomized versus fixed time schedules for quality control procedures. Clin Chem 2007;53:575–80.
11. Parvin CA. Estimating the performance characteristics of quality-control procedures when error persists until detection. Clin Chem 1991;37:1720–4.
12. Parvin CA. Assessing the impact of the frequency of quality control testing on the quality of reported patient results. Clin Chem 2008;54:2049–54.
13. Yundt-Pacheco JC. The impact of QC frequency on patient results. MLO Med Lab Obs 2008;40:26–7.
14. Cembrowski GS, Carey RN. Quality control procedures. In: Laboratory quality management. Chicago: ASCP Press; 1989. p. 59–79.
15. Parvin CA. Comparing the power of quality-control rules to detect persistent systematic error. Clin Chem 1992;38:358–63.
16. Parvin CA. Comparing the power of quality-control rules to detect persistent increases in random error. Clin Chem 1992;38:364–9.
17. Parvin CA, Kuchipudi LS, Yundt-Pacheco JC. Should I repeat my 1:2s QC rejection? Clin Chem 2012;58:925–9.
18. Parvin CA. New insight into the comparative power of quality-control rules that use control observations within a single analytical run. Clin Chem 1993;39:440–7.
19. Parvin CA, Gronowski AM. Effect of analytical run length on quality-control (QC) performance and the QC planning process. Clin Chem 1997;43:2149–54.
20. Yundt-Pacheco JC. Instrument reliability and QC frequency: a cautionary tale. MLO Med Lab Obs 2009;41:28.

Integrated Quality Control

Implementation and Validation of Instrument Function Checks and Procedural Controls for a Cartridge-Based Point-of-Care System for Critical Care Analysis

Paul D'Orazio, PhD*, Sohrab Mansouri, PhD

KEYWORDS

- Critical care analyzers • Integrated quality control • Failure pattern recognition
- Risk management

KEY POINTS

- Risk management principles are being applied to best control all phases of the laboratory testing process (preanalytical, analytical, and postanalytical).
- Instruments for critical care analysis include a high degree of self-diagnostics, aimed primarily at recognizing mechanical and electrical system failures.
- As critical care analyzers are being used increasingly in point-of-care (POC) locations, integrated quality control (QC) systems are being developed to make QC an automatic, ongoing process and to simplify QC for operators at POC locations.
- Integrated QC consists of statistical QC using onboard reference solutions and failure pattern recognition aimed at controlling known failure modes within the analytical stage of the testing process.

INTRODUCTION

The growing use of clinical analyzers in point-of-care (POC) environments, by nonlaboratory personnel, has placed increased demands on instrument manufacturers to develop systems with enhanced ease-of-use, low maintenance, and simplicity in quality control (QC). Instruments for blood gas analysis were among the first clinical analyzers to make the transition from the central laboratory to POC environments as a result of the time-sensitive nature of these tests in delivery of patient care. A survey

Research and Development, Instrumentation Laboratory, 180 Hartwell Road, Bedford, MA 01730, USA
* Corresponding author.
E-mail address: pdorazio@ilww.com

Clin Lab Med 33 (2013) 89–109
http://dx.doi.org/10.1016/j.cll.2012.11.001 labmed.theclinics.com
0272-2712/13/$ – see front matter © 2013 Elsevier Inc. All rights reserved.

published by Enterprise Analysis Corporation (Stamford, CT) in 2011[1] concluded that 72% of institutions were running blood gases at POC, surpassed only by blood glucose testing. Although systems for critical care testing (pH, blood gases, electrolytes, and metabolites) have evolved from maintenance-intensive, classic benchtop units to cartridge-based, handheld and portable systems, the goal of a QC program has not changed. A QC program should be designed to evaluate the complete analytical process used to generate test results, in terms of ability to detect failure or to reduce probability of failure. Failure is defined as a perturbation in accuracy or precision of a test system outside performance claims, potentially resulting in reporting of patient results containing errors of clinical significance.

The classic approach to QC requires an operator to assay commercially available control materials (often referred to as surrogate samples), based on time schedules and concentration levels mandated by regulatory agencies. Analytical results outside statistically determined limits may indicate the presence of a problem. Instrument self-diagnostics may or may not flag the source of the problem, leaving the user to troubleshoot the problem until analyte concentrations recover to acceptable limits. Because this type of QC is not continuous, errors in system performance taking place between discrete testing of surrogate samples may go undetected. Meanwhile, patient samples continue to be assayed, increasing the likelihood of reporting erroneous results.

Most modern critical care analyzers include a high degree of instrument self-diagnostics, for example, system integrity checks to ensure proper functioning of mechanical components, such as pumps and valves, detection of occlusions within the fluidic system, and checks of the electronics and microprocessor communications. Some of these features are listed in **Box 1**. However, these hardware checks do not monitor the key part of the analytical process: the sensing of an analyte concentration in a patient sample.

Box 1
Examples of hardware integrity checks built into systems for critical care testing

System Fluidic Checks

- Reagent flow and volume
- Sample flow and volume
- Sampling device operation
- Expiration dates of reagents

Electronic and Mechanical Checks

- Temperature measurement of sensing system
- Electrical signal transmission from sensors
- Analog/digital electronic calibration verification
- Pump, valve, and motor movements
- Microprocessor communications
- Optical system checks (for instruments including oximetry measurements)

Corrective Actions

- Error message displayed to user
- System or user initiated corrective action
- System operation halted for unrecoverable failure

HOW IS QC EVOLVING ON THE NEW POC CRITICAL CARE ANALYZERS?

Handheld and portable systems for critical care testing have expanded test menus, using miniaturized electrochemical sensors for blood gases, electrolytes, and metabolites, and the capability to measure hemoglobin and fractional components of hemoglobin using optical-sensing technology. In many systems, sensors and reagents are contained within disposable measurement cartridges. These cartridges are used to assay a fixed number of samples, ranging from 1 (single-use cartridge) to several hundred, over a period of up to 4 weeks. Internal troubleshooting of sensor malfunctions, reagent deterioration, and cartridge fluidics by the user is not possible. This cartridge-based approach reduces demands for operator intervention, but places increased demands on the instrument to carry out self-diagnostics and corrective actions. The following are examples of types of QC systems, developed by manufacturers and already used for several years in newer cartridge-based analyzers for POC testing.

Electronic QC

Electronic (EQC) was developed specifically for single-use testing systems because QC cannot be performed on the same test cartridge used to assay a patient sample. This approach uses a simulator, either built into the analytical system or a separate device, in place of a test cartridge to monitor the electronic components of the analytical system. EQC has the advantage of being simple, quick, and inexpensive, with little dependence on operator skill. However, EQC monitors only a portion of the analytical system and does not monitor sensing reactions or sampling-related functions. Single-use cartridges are typically tested with surrogate samples only when a new manufactured lot of test cartridges is introduced, before being accepted for clinical use. A limited series of preset diagnostics is performed on introduction of each test cartridge, from validating the reagent to monitoring the quantity of the sample, and a cartridge may be rejected for gross failure before or during analysis of a patient sample.

Automatic QC

This QC system uses surrogate samples, which may be packaged within a disposable cartridge, separate from the sample measurement cartridge, or included within the same cartridge used to assay patient samples. Automatic QC (auto QC) is similar to ampouled QC but packaged differently and is more convenient. The fluidic path for QC materials is through the patient sample entry port of the cartridge. Assay of the surrogate samples is performed based on a user-selected schedule. The assessment of control status follows traditional QC with control limits of 2 or 3 standard deviation (SD) limits. On failure to properly recover an analyte concentration in the surrogate sample, some automatic corrective actions may be initiated. These actions include extra flushing of the sensor cartridge fluid pathways, sensor recalibration, and parameter shutoff for persistent QC failure. Auto QC has the advantage of requiring no user intervention for required QC testing, but QC testing is still discrete, and errors that occur between assays of the QC materials may go undetected.

Continuous (Integrated) QC

The impetus for development of integrated QC has been 2-fold: first, to simplify QC processes for increased acceptance of systems in POC environments where testing is performed by nonlaboratory personnel, and second, to make QC an ongoing, continuous process, with the goal of minimizing risk of reporting erroneous patient data. Mechanisms, integrated into the design of a device, have been developed to carry out continuous system QC. These automated internal checks are capable of monitoring the quality of a raw sensor signal each time an onboard reagent or patient sample is assayed, to indicate if the system is performing within expected limits. The system may also check for certain patterns in the sensor signal, which indicate the integrity of a patient sample (eg, presence of a blood clot, interfering substance or air bubble lodged on a sensor). If a situation outside acceptable limits is detected, a corrective action specific to the source of the error is initiated. The corrective actions include: extra system flushing if the presence of a clot is detected, accelerated QC checks if the presence of an interfering substance is detected, or correcting for sensor drift if no specific malfunction can be detected. If the corrective action is not successful, a sensor may be temporarily disabled and re-enabled at a later time if the situation is determined to be corrected. The major advantage of continuous QC is the performance testing of the entire analytical system with measurement of each patient sample, without operator intervention.

Recently, the Clinical and Laboratory Standards Institute (CLSI) published document Evaluation Protocol 23-A (EP23-A), *Laboratory Quality Control Based on Risk Management*.[2] Although risk management is a new concept for managing quality within the clinical laboratory, manufacturers of instruments for in vitro diagnostics have been required for several years to conduct risk analysis of new devices under ISO (International Organization for Standardization) 14971 as part of their design control process.[3] The concept of integrated QC continues to develop using this risk analysis approach, in which manufacturers have developed checks and controls, built into their diagnostic devices, for reducing the probability of failure or increasing probability of detecting failure of critical components involved in the testing process. In a properly designed system, failure detection takes place before erroneous patient data are reported.

In this article, an example is presented of the process to develop and validate instrument function checks and procedural controls as part of an integrated QC system implemented by 1 manufacturer. This example is specific to measurement of pH, blood gases, electrolytes, glucose, lactate, and hematocrit in a cartridge-based critical care analyzer designed for POC testing, the GEM Premier 3000 (Instrumentation Laboratory, Bedford, MA) and its onboard system for quality management (Intelligent Quality Management [iQM]).

IDENTIFYING SOURCES OF ERROR AND METHODS OF CONTROL FOR A CARTRIDGE-BASED CRITICAL CARE ANALYZER

Medical errors resulting from laboratory medicine are recognized as originating from preanalytical, analytical, and postanalytical phases of the testing process, with error rates distributed among the 3 stages, as summarized in **Fig. 1**.[4,5] A study by Carraro and Plebani in 2007,[6] 10 years after their original 1997 study,[5] showed an overall reduction in errors in stat laboratory testing over a 10-year period, because of increased awareness of sources of errors, but with distribution of errors among preanalytical, analytical, and postanalytical phases equivalent to their original study and in agreement with **Fig. 1**: preanalytical (62%), analytical (15%), postanalytical (23%). Clinical laboratories have accepted the benefits of statistical QC for some time; however, statistical QC detects the presence of errors primarily during the analytical phase of the testing process, although, as shown, most errors take place during the preanalytical and postanalytical phases. A more comprehensive system to monitor all phases of the testing process is needed. Development of QC plans in accordance with CLSI EP23-A and application of risk management principles provides an approach to address this need.

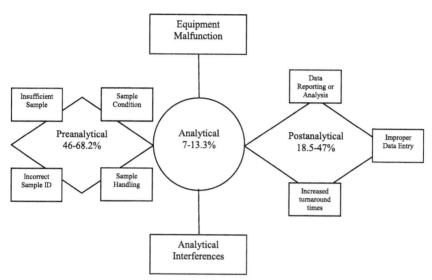

Fig. 1. Types and rates of errors at the 3 stages of the laboratory testing process: preanalytical, analytical, and postanalytical. (*Adapted from* Kalra J. Medical errors: impact on clinical laboratories and other critical areas. Clin Biochem 2004;37:1055; with permission.)

The first step of risk management is to understand sources of error during each stage of the testing process with the goal of designing integrated QC features to detect errors and prevent or reduce their occurrence. A manufacturer may carry out an evaluation of sources of error such as that shown in **Table 1**, which lists failure modes for each stage of the testing process (preanalytical, analytical, and postanalytical), which may result in reporting of erroneous patient data using the example of a cartridge-based critical care analyzer. Listed for each failure mode are methods for detecting or reducing probability of failure using external QC, integrated QC, and other methods such as operator training and laboratory-implemented monitors. Definitions of external QC and integrated QC used in **Table 1** are consistent with those in CLSI EP23-A.

External QC (Also Called Intralaboratory QC)

External QC is periodic measurement of stable QC materials, designed to mimic as much as possible the analytical behavior of patient samples. The use of QC samples to monitor a measuring system involves establishing the mean and SD for the specific QC sample lot and determining statistical limits that identify unacceptable changes in performance of the measuring system.

Integrated QC (Also Called Controls Built into the Measuring System)

Integrated QC includes: (a) QC samples built into reagent packs or unit-use reagent systems, measured automatically by the analytical system (results are compared against statistically predetermined limits similar to external QC samples), (b) detection mechanisms to monitor critical functions related to the measuring system including automatic correction of malfunctions, reporting of error messages to the user, and blocking reporting of test results until the malfunction is corrected, and (c) calibration checks to monitor and correct drift in the measuring system before patient samples are assayed.

Table 1
Failure modes and methods for detecting or reducing probability of failure in a cartridge-based critical care analyzer

Failure Mode	External QC	Integrated QC	Operator Training and Laboratory-Implemented Monitors
		Method for Detecting or Reducing Probability of Failure	
Preanalytical Stage			
Incorrect sampling site selection and preparation	N/A	N/A	Training on appropriate selection and preparation of site for sample collection using resources such as CLSI H03-A6, H11-A4, and C46-A2
Incorrect sample acquisition from an arterial catheter	N/A	N/A	Training and competency assessment on appropriate technique for drawing from an indwelling line using resources such as CLSI H11-A4
Incorrect technique for capillary sample collection	N/A	N/A	Training and competency assessment on appropriate technique for collecting capillary samples using resources such as CLSI H04-A6
Incorrect sample collection device	N/A	N/A	Training on use of collection devices appropriate for blood gas measurements (ie, heparinized syringe or capillary). Ensure that only correct devices are available for sample collection
Incomplete sample draw	N/A	System may report "insufficient sample volume" in cases of short draw, resulting in less than minimum sample for analysis. Sample is rejected and message displayed to user	Train operators of the consequences of underfilling collection device. Competency assessment includes observation of specimen collection
Improper sample mixing	N/A	System may include automated devices at front end to assure adequate sample mixing	Train operators in proper sample mixing to assure sample homogeneity and to avoid clot formation. Competency assessment includes observation of specimen mixing

Incorrect lancet for capillary sample collection	N/A	N/A	Train operators to use appropriate lancet device with appropriate depth of puncture using resources such as CLSI H04-A6
Air in syringe/sample exposed to air	N/A	Aspiration of air from syringe into the system may be flagged as an error. Sample rejected and no results reported. Message displayed to user	Train operators in appropriate sample collection technique to prevent air in syringe and to eliminate sample exposure to air, especially if pneumatic tube transport is used. Resources such as CLSI C46-A2 may be used
Samples incorrectly stored on ice	N/A	N/A	Train operators on importance of not icing samples before testing, especially if plastic syringes are used (Po_2 results may be falsely increased and K^+ falsely decreased). Resources such as CLSI C46-A2 and H11-A4 may be used
Hemolyzed samples	N/A	N/A	Train operators in sample collection and handling technique, highlighting how to prevent cell lysis. Samples with elevated K^+ should be suspected for hemolysis
Hemodiluted samples	N/A	Extremely diluted samples, with less than minimum electrical conductivity, may be rejected by system, no results reported and message displayed to user	Train operators as appropriate (such as those who work with cardiopulmonary bypass solutions) on hemodilution interferences
Blood clots in sample	N/A	If blood clots are present in sample, instrument may attempt to clear the clot or provide message that unable to move sample or that clots have been detected. No sample results are reported. Clot catchers may be engineered into the system front end to prevent aspiration of clots	Train operators to collect samples using devices containing correct heparin levels. Train operators to collect, mix, and handle sample in a manner that prevents clot formation. Use manufacturer's training information and CLSI C46-A2 as resources

(continued on next page)

Table 1
(continued)

	Method for Detecting or Reducing Probability of Failure		
Failure Mode	External QC	Integrated QC	Operator Training and Laboratory-Implemented Monitors
Excessive time delay between receiving and testing sample	N/A	Instrument data management software may identify time difference between sample collection and measurement, and presents message to user	Train operators on maximum amount of time sample can remain in collection device before analysis, using resources such as CLSI C46-A2
Overfill of cartridge (specific to unit-use devices)	N/A	Instrument identifies when cartridge is overfilled, rejects cartridge, and presents message to user	Train operators on sample filling procedure, including fill mark level on cartridge. Information included in manufacturer's training literature
Insufficient sample volume aspirated or applied to cartridge	N/A	Instrument identifies when insufficient sample has been applied, automatically rejects sample, does not report results, and displays message to user	Train operators on how to correctly apply samples to system using manufacturer's training information
Incorrect ptient identification	N/A	Instrument requires positive patient identification, and device blocks operator from testing unless positive identification established	Two patient identifiers should be required. Operators should be trained on proper sample identification and labeling using resources such as CLSI C46-A2 and H03-A6
Analytical Stage			
Electronic component failure	System may not accept external QC if electronic component failure detected	Instrument has electronic self-checks that abort testing process or shut down analyzer if electronic component failure or power interruption is detected (see **Box 1**)	Train operators that instrument has self-checks that abort testing process if electronic component failure detected. Information included in manufacturer's system manual
Mechanical component failure	System may not accept external QC if mechanical component failure detected	Instrument has mechanical self-checks (eg, pump, motor movement) that abort testing process or shut down analyzer if failure detected (see **Box 1**)	Train operators that instrument has self-checks that abort testing process if mechanical component failure detected. Information included in manufacturer's system manual

Software failures	System may not accept external QC if software failure detected	Instrument checks software version, recognizes outdated or invalid software or software errors, prevents testing, and provides instructions for next action	Train operators that instrument recognizes outdated or invalid software and software errors. Information included in manufacturer's system manual
Air aspirated into system	N/A	Instrument has electronic air detection that rejects samples containing air, does not report result, and presents message to user	Train operators in appropriate specimen collection technique to prevent air in sample and to expel air from sample as needed. Resources such as CLSI C46-A2 may be used
Sample contamination or carryover	External QC may detect sample contamination or carryover by failure to recover correct values, depending on timing of material assay relative to sample	Onboard QC materials may detect sample contamination or carryover, prevent reporting of results, and alert user. Intervention (cartridge replacement for multiuse cartridge) or instrument service may be required	Operator should question results that seem discrepant. Repeat sample analysis if possible
Sensor failure	External QC may detect sensor failure by failure to recover correct values, depending on timing of material assay relative to sample	Onboard QC materials or electronic integrity checks may detect sensor failure. Sensor may be disabled and no results reported for that analyte. Intervention (cartridge replacement) or instrument maintenance may be required	N/A
Sensor drift	External QC may detect sensor drift by failure to recover correct values, depending on timing of material assay relative to sample	Onboard QC materials may detect sensor drift and question sample results. Automatic corrective action (sensor recalibration) may be initiated	N/A
Hematocrit interference	N/A	N/A	Review product literature to familiarize operators with manufacturer's claims for hematocrit interference

(continued on next page)

Table 1 (continued)			
	Method for Detecting or Reducing Probability of Failure		
Failure Mode	**External QC**	**Integrated QC**	**Operator Training and Laboratory-Implemented Monitors**
Chemical interferences (endogenous or exogenous substances) present in sample	External QC may detect failure if interfering substance produces hysteresis or permanent damage to a sensor, depending on timing of material assay relative to sample	Instrument software checks may flag presence of certain interfering substances if a characteristic fingerprint is left on a sensor signal. System attempts to recover sensor function or disable sensor in case of irreversible damage	Review product literature to familiarize operators with manufacturer's claims for interfering substances. If sample results seem questionable, consult patient history for any drugs, and so forth that may produce interference. CLSI C46-A2 and EP7-A2 may be used as resources
Clot formation in analyzer	External QC may detect failure if clot produces perturbation of sensor signal resulting in incorrect results, or blockage of fluidics	Instrument software checks may flag presence of clot if a characteristic fingerprint is left on a sensor signal or if clot blocks fluidic flow. System may attempt to clear clot or disable sensor or prompt user to replace cartridge in case of irreversible damage	Train operators to collect samples using devices containing correct heparin levels. Train operators to collect, mix, and handle sample in a manner that prevents clot formation. Use manufacturer's training information and CLSI C46-A2 as resources
Improper reagent shipping conditions	Test 2 levels of liquid QC for each lot of reagents in use or for each new cartridge used in analyzer. Results should be within manufacturer's stated ranges for acceptance of new material	Shipment sent with single-use temperature strip to detect thermal stress. Temperature strip result must be read and recorded. If out of range, contact manufacturer for further instruction. On introduction of new reagent lot or cartridge, system may not allow assay of patient samples until 2 levels of external QC have been tested and produce results within manufacturer's stated ranges	Verify integrity of shipped materials on arrival. Train operators on proper use of temperature strip results and any needed follow-up activity

Improper reagent storage conditions	Test 2 levels of liquid QC for each lot of reagents in use or for each new cartridge used in analyzer. Results should be within manufacturer's stated ranges for acceptance of new material	On introduction of a new reagent cartridge, system may not allow assay of patient samples until 2 levels of external QC have been tested and produce results within manufacturer's stated ranges	Store consumables per manufacturer's recommendations. Provide refrigerator temperature monitoring program for storage of reagents/consumables requiring refrigeration. For consumables requiring ambient storage, ensure that ambient temperature and storage time are within manufacturer's recommendations
Reagents used past expiration date	N/A	Instrument identifies when cartridge is expired, automatically rejects cartridge under these conditions, and presents message to user	Train operators on importance of and location of product expiration dates
Improper QC material shipping conditions	N/A	Shipment sent with single-use temperature strip to detect thermal stress. Temperature strip result must be read and recorded. If out of range, material should not be used. Contact manufacturer for further instruction	Verify integrity of shipped materials on arrival. Train operators on proper use of temperature strip results and any needed follow-up activity
Improper QC material storage conditions	N/A	N/A	Store QC materials per manufacturer's recommendations. Provide refrigerator temperature monitoring program for storage of QC materials requiring refrigeration. For QC materials requiring ambient storage, ensure that ambient temperature and storage time are within manufacturer's recommendations

(continued on next page)

Table 1
(continued)

	Method for Detecting or Reducing Probability of Failure		
Failure Mode	External QC	Integrated QC	Operator Training and Laboratory-Implemented Monitors
QC material used past expiration date	N/A	Instrument identifies when controls are past expiration date, automatically rejects control testing, and presents message to user	Train operators how to locate QC material expiration dates and not to use expired QC materials
Incorrect QC material preparation and use	N/A	N/A	Train operators in preparation and use of QC materials per manufacturer's instructions. Equilibrate ampoule for required amount of time at temperature specified by manufacturer. Sample from bottom of ampoule, and use each ampoule for only 1 determination
Inadequate instrument maintenance	External QC may detect error if improper instrument maintenance results in failure or malfunction of a critical analytical component (eg, salt solution on system electronics)	POC systems are designed to require little or no maintenance. Failure of a critical analytical component is detected by onboard system checks	Train operators in required instrument maintenance as described in manufacturer's documentation
Improper instrument shutdown	External QC may detect error if improper instrument shutdown results in failure or malfunction of a critical analytical component	Onscreen prompts guide operator through proper instrument shutdown. If improper shutdown results in failure or malfunction of a critical analytical component, system checks detect failure during instrument restart	Train operators in proper instrument shutdown procedure, as described in manufacturer's training literature
Improper handling of cartridge	If mishandling results in damage to cartridge analytical functionality, external QC materials may detect the failure	Instrument has detection capability of cartridges damaged by mishandling. System automatically rejects cartridge under these conditions and presents message to user	Train operators on how to handle and store cartridges per manufacturer's instructions

	External QC	Internal system check	Corrective action
Improper insertion of cartridge	Cartridges not inserted properly may result in failure to recover expected results for external QCs	Onscreen prompts guide operator through proper cartridge insertion. Instrument has detection system for cartridges that are not inserted properly, automatically rejects cartridges under this condition, and presents message to user	Train operators to insert cartridge per manufacturer's instructions
Electromagnetic interference	External QC may fail to recover correct values if electromagnetic interference affects stability of measuring system	System checks detect instability of measuring system produced by electromagnetic interference	Instrument placement in laboratory should be in conformance with manufacturer's recommendations
Improper line voltage or power interruption	External QC may fail to recover correct values if improper line voltage or power interruption affects stability of measuring system	System checks detect mechanical, electrical, or sensor failures produced by improper line voltage or power interruption. System displays message to user and prevents assay of patient samples	Connect system to electrical service with proper voltage per manufacturer's recommendations. Information included in system manual. Uninterruptable power supply or line filter should be used if recommended by manufacturer
Ambient temperature outside instrument specification	External QC may fail to recover correct values if ambient temperature outside instrument specification produces thermal instability of measuring system	Instrument detects measuring system temperature out of range. System displays message to user and prevents assay of patient samples	Train operators on monitoring of ambient temperature for conformance with instrument specifications
Ambient humidity outside instrument specification	N/A	System checks detect mechanical or electrical failures produced by high or low humidity. System displays message to user and prevents assay of patient samples	Train operators on monitoring of ambient humidity for conformance with instrument specifications
Barometric pressure outside instrument specification	External QC may fail to recover correct values if barometric pressure outside instrument specification produces incorrect gas tensions in calibrators	If system contains internal barometer, system checks detect barometric pressure outside operating limits. System displays message to user and prevents assay of patient samples	Train operators on monitoring of barometric pressure for conformance with instrument specifications. Information included in manufacturer's system manual

(continued on next page)

Table 1
(continued)

Failure Mode	Method for Detecting or Reducing Probability of Failure		
	External QC	Integrated QC	Operator Training and Laboratory-Implemented Monitors
Environmental dust and debris	External QC may fail to recover correct values if dust or debris damages electrical or mechanical components	Air filters guard against dust and debris entering system. If dust or debris enters system, mechanical and electrical system checks may detect damage, display message to user, and prevent assay of patient samples	Train operators on importance of clean laboratory environment. If dust or debris is unavoidable in certain POC locations, instrument should be placed to minimize chance of dust or debris entering system. Information included in manufacturer's system manual
Postanalytical Stage			
Connectivity software failure transmits no data or corrupted data to Laboratory Information System/Hospital Information System	N/A	Instrument detects failure to complete a data transmission and provides message to user	Institution's information technology department should ensure instrument software compatibility with Laboratory Information System/Hospital Information System and compliance with requirements for connectivity, in accordance with manufacturer's recommendations
Failure to report critical values	N/A	Instrument flags patient data outside preset reference ranges	Operators should be trained in the importance of confirming and calling in critical values
Failure to detect erroneous result, which may not be flagged or prevented by integrated QC	N/A	Instrument may provide patient data tracking, allowing correlation between patient condition and test results	Train operators to question results that seem implausible. Conduct repeat sample analysis on a different system if possible

Abbreviation: N/A, not applicable.

Review of **Table 1** indicates that neither external nor integrated QC, taken individually, is a complete form of QC. A combination of statistical QC based on assay of surrogate samples and integrated function checks and procedural controls aimed at controlling known weak areas of the testing process is the most effective form of QC. The importance of operator training and other laboratory-implemented monitors, to complement the other forms of QC, cannot be overlooked in managing risk during the entire testing process.

DESIGN AND VALIDATION OF STATISTICAL QC FOR THE GEM PREMIER 3000

The GEM Premier 3000 is a cartridge-based analyzer for measurement of pH, blood gases, electrolytes (Na^+, K^+, Ca^{2+}), glucose, lactate, and hematocrit at POC. An integrated quality management system for the instrument (iQM), was introduced in 2002. A test cartridge is a closed, self-contained analytical system including all components required for sample analysis (sensors, process control solutions [PCSs], sample probe, valves for sample selection, tubing, and waste bag). No change affecting performance can be introduced to the cartridge analytical components during cartridge use-life, so the cartridge use-life may be considered a single analytical run as defined by CLSI Document C24-A3.[7]

Installation of a new cartridge involves user verification of performance using 2 levels of external controls before patient samples can be analyzed. After successful verification using the external controls, cartridge performance is monitored at various frequencies throughout the use-life by analysis of 3 onboard reference solutions called PCS A, B, and C, containing different concentrations of the analytes of interest.

- PCS A is analyzed every 4 hours.
- PCS B is analyzed every 30 minutes, or after every patient sample.
  - During instrument idle time, PCS B is introduced every 30 minutes, and sensor signals are monitored every 30 seconds.
- PCS C is analyzed every 24 hours.

Drift limits for PCS A, B, and C were characterized from measurements of each material using cartridge data. Statistical control methods were then used to develop probabilities for error detection (P_{ed}) and false rejection (P_{fr}) and to calculate time required to detect an error.[8]

Time required to detect an error condition for each channel on the GEM Premier 3000 analyzer, using PCS A and B, has been analyzed and reported using data from 24 different test cartridges with an average of 85 measurements of PCS A and 725 measurements of PCS B per cartridge.[8] The overall process for arriving at time to error detection was as follows:

1. Total allowable error for each analyte was defined based on Clinical Laboratory Improvement Amendments proficiency testing criteria.[9]
2. Precision was measured for each analyte.
3. Sigma metric was calculated for each analyte (total allowable error/measured precision).
4. Statistical control limit was calculated for each analyte (specified drift limit/measured precision). P_{ed} and P_{fr} were determined from standard tables of normal probability distribution, as described in Ref.[8]

Note: drift limit for each analyte in step 4 may be optimized based on what is practically achievable for a measurement technology and to maximize P_{ed} and minimize P_{fr}.

5. P_{ed} was used to calculate the average number of PCS measurements needed to detect a problem for a particular analyte ($1/P_{ed}$). Multiplying number of PCS measurements by time interval for analysis of each PCS was then used to calculate time to error detection.

Times to error detection using PCS A and B is shown in **Table 2** for each analyte reported by the system. The data demonstrate that during periods of analysis of patient samples, 1 measurement of PCS B (sampled every 3 minutes when measuring patient samples) is sufficient to detect an error condition for pH, P_{CO_2}, P_{O_2}, K^+, Ca^{2+}, lactate, and hematocrit. For Na^+ and glucose, 10 and 7 minutes, respectively, are required to detect an error condition using PCS B. The higher times to error detection for these analytes are largely caused by less-than-optimal precision for these 2 sensors. Nevertheless, times to error detection using the onboard PCSs are superior to detection times using traditional externally assayed QC materials, which typically are analyzed once per 8-hour work shift.

DESIGN AND VALIDATION OF FAILURE PATTERN RECOGNITION FOR THE GEM PREMIER 3000

Enhancements to a QC procedure can be established through understanding of specific failure modes during the preanalytical, analytical, and postanalytical phases of the testing process. In particular, during the analytical phase, sensing related functions such as those listed in **Table 1** may be affected by patient blood samples containing interfering substances, blood clots, and so forth, resulting in specific patterns to a sensor signal, which indicate a failure mode. These failure modes are not detectable by external QC unless the QC material is assayed immediately after the patient sample and unexpected results are obtained.

Given the variety of testing performed in a typical health care facility with a particular measuring system, detailed examination of past end-user data anomalies provides a means for identifying their root cause. This methodology of understanding failure modes through postexamination of available end-user data can be achieved only if the measuring system is capable of collecting adequate information. The GEM Premier 3000 is an example of a measuring system that collects large amounts of data during every cartridge operation, including raw sensor outputs, all fluidic, mechanical, and electrical checks, and all measurement results, including samples, calibrations, and drifts. Years of investigating these data provided a list of distinct patterns associated with specific failure modes. These patterns were subsequently verified through in-house testing by recreating the failure and verifying the pattern. This methodology provided the basis for developing failure pattern recognition (FPR) checks to be incorporated in the analyzer software for active and continuous detection of known weaknesses of the analytical system. FPR allows identification of failures that otherwise would be undetected by existing internal checks.[10] Two

Table 2
Average time to error detection for available analytes on the GEM Premier 3000 using PCS A and B

pH	P_{CO_2}	P_{O_2}	Na^+	K^+	Ca^{2+}	Glucose	Lactate	Hematocrit
PCS A (h)								
4.27	8.33	4.11	10.2	4.00	4.06	4.06	7.87	Not applicable
PCS B (min) (sampled every 3 min during periods of patient sample analysis)								
3	3	3	10	3	3	7	3	3

examples follow of FPR consisting of distinct patterns in sensor outputs that represent certain malfunctions in the analytical system.

Microclot-Related Failures

Small blood clots or fibrin strands can adhere to a sensor surface and induce a change in sensor characteristics such as sluggish response or sensitivity change. This change in sensor characteristics generates distinct response patterns that are used by FPR for detecting microclots. Using a Po_2 sensor as an example, **Fig. 2** shows patterns in signals generated by the sensor when analyzing PCSs A and B to detect presence of a clot on the sensor and to verify that actions undertaken by the system have successfully removed the clot from the sensor. In routine operation, PCS B (Po_2 = 180 mm Hg) is analyzed after every blood sample, and PCS A (Po_2 = 118 mm Hg) is analyzed every 4 hours during cartridge operation. After analysis of a blood sample, a negative shift in PCS B result away from the expected value triggers immediate analysis of PCS A. A positive shift in PCS A is used to confirm presence of a clot. After confirmation, the system initiates vigorous rinsing of the sensor with an onboard surfactant-containing solution. Successful removal of the clot is indicated by return of the PCS B and A results to the expected values (top and bottom arrows, respectively, in **Fig. 2**). If the expected PCS B and A values are not recovered, the sensor is disabled and is no longer available for reporting sample results. The system may attempt to restore sensor function at a later time.

Interference from Charged Lipophilic Compounds

FPR flags have been developed for interference by charged lipophilic compounds with the ion-selective electrodes. Benzalkonium is a cationic disinfecting agent coated on the surface of indwelling catheters as a biocide. When a blood sample is drawn from a newly placed indwelling catheter, some benzalkonium may be extracted into the sample. During sample analysis, benzalkonium partitions into the sensing membranes of polyvinyl chloride (PVC)-based cation-selective electrodes, producing an interfering signal. Because of the lipophilic nature of benzalkonium, the ion is slow to extract from the ion-selective sensing membranes, producing a slow return to the sensor baseline.

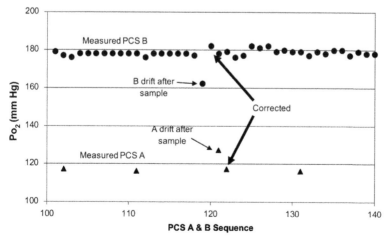

Fig. 2. Patterns in signals generated by a Po_2 sensor when analyzing PCS A and PCS B to detect presence of a clot on the sensor and recovery of sensor function after the clot has been removed from the sensor. Arrows indicate measurements of PCSs B and A with results returning to the expected values.

FPR for the GEM Premier 3000 incorporates pattern checks for the presence of benzalkonium in a sample. **Fig. 3** shows the pattern check using measured concentrations of Na^+ and Ca^{2+} in PCS B. After exposure of the sensors to a blood sample containing benzalkonium, the sensors show an increased measurement for PCS B, indicating that the preceding blood sample likely contained a positive interference because of benzalkonium. The increase in PCS B baseline after sample exposure for both the Na^+ and Ca^{2+} sensors is used to confirm presence of benzalkonium in the sample. A message is displayed to the user indicating likely interference by benzalkonium on the Na^+ and Ca^{2+} results of the preceding sample. Lipophilic cations other than benzalkonium in patient blood samples are rare; however, similar FPR flags have been included in the GEM Premier 3000 for interference from lipophilic anions with various PVC-based sensors. Because there are many lipophilic anions (eg, drugs) that may interfere, patterns from lipophilic anions are unspecified as chemical species.

Similar GEM Premier 3000 FPR checks have been developed to address other known analytical failure modes, for example, those related to malfunctions of specific sensors as well as presence of an air bubble over a sensor during sample measurement, leading to a distinct deviation from a normal sensor response pattern.

Effectiveness of FPR error detection was investigated using existing end-user data files for the GEM Premier 3000. The investigation focused on 79 field complaints for failure to pass traditional QC, after cartridge installation and during use-life, from domestic US accounts of approximately 7000 cartridge shipments. Cartridge data for these QC discrepancies were analyzed and matched with proposed FPR checks to test if the root cause of failure could be determined. The results are summarized as follows:

- Sixty-eight had microclot patterns
- Six showed sensor failure patterns
- Five had no identifiable pattern

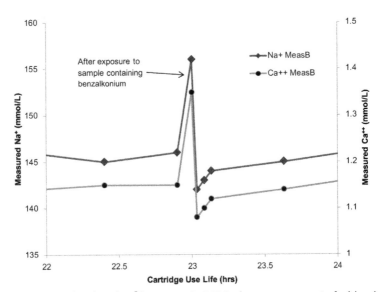

Fig. 3. Patterns for of Na^+ and Ca^{2+} recovery in PCS B after measurement of a blood sample containing benzalkonium. Arrow indicates elevated measurements of PCS B after exposure of the sensors to a sample containing benzalkonium.

This analysis indicates that FPR was able to detect malfunction in 74 of 79 reported QC failures. For the clot-related failures, FPR would have flagged the failure immediately after the sample that caused the malfunction, whereas the user became aware of the problem up to many hours later because of inability to recover correct QC values. No obvious malfunction was detected in the data from 5 cartridges that FPR did not flag but had reported QC failures. All system parameters were found within specifications. No anomaly was noted in the blood results, and the QC failure was marginal and at 1 level only. It was concluded that 5 reported QC failures were not representing a serious cartridge malfunction, which could have resulted in reporting of erroneous patient data, and were likely false-positive results.

The field data analysis showed effectiveness of FPR in identifying known cartridge malfunctions. In addition, the active and real-time aspects of iQM allow for immediate error detection and correction, enhancing the QC capabilities of the analyzer.

USER EVALUATION OF STATISTICAL QC AND FPR FOR THE GEM PREMIER 3000

The performance claims of statistical QC for the GEM Premier 3000 using analysis of onboard PCSs as part of the iQM system were evaluated at 4 clinical sites while analyzing approximately 10,550 patient samples.[11] A total of 35 measurement cartridges were installed in GEM Premier 3000 analyzers at the 4 sites. Systems were operated by technicians, nurses, respiratory therapists, perfusionists, and physicians, who received training on instrument setup and operation. Data using the onboard PCS materials were used to calculate average time to error detection for each analyte and compared with data obtained from analysis of traditional external controls on GEM Premier 3000 systems operated simultaneously at 2 of the clinical sites. Average time to error detection using data from analysis of PCS B on the systems with iQM was estimated at 3 minutes for all analytes except sodium (17.3 minutes), glucose (11.4 minutes), and lactate (5.9 minutes). These estimated error detection times are in good agreement with those found earlier during design and validation of statistical QC of iQM on the GEM Premier 3000.[8] The average sigma value for Na^+ on the GEM Premier 3000 with iQM was only 2.7, indicating that the Na^+ sensor requires more frequent monitoring. Because PCS B is measured so frequently, the average time to error detection for sodium was 17.3 minutes, even with a lower-than-optimum sigma value. This time to error detection is superior to systems running external controls, in which controls may be run only once during an 8-hour shift, and errors occurring between analyses of external controls may go undetected.

The short time to error detection by iQM results from frequent monitoring and high precision observed for measurements of the onboard PCS B. Sigma values measured during the end-user evaluation of iQM were 6 or greater for all analytes except sodium (sigma = 2.7). In contrast, only 15 of 26 sigma values on 2 GEM Premier 3000 systems running external controls were 6 or greater, because of more imprecision for analysis of external controls (sigma = total allowable error/SD). The improvement in sigma for the systems with iQM, especially for blood gases and pH, is partly because internal PCSs are not susceptible to user handling of external controls.

It was concluded during the multisite evaluation that FPR is the most important benefit of the iQM process. About 1 in 200 samples were flagged for some type of analytical problem, as summarized in **Table 3**. For microclots, the affected sensors were disabled while the system attempted to remove the clot. Of the 14 microclots observed during this evaluation, all but one were cleared within 1 hour, and one was cleared after 10 hours. These types of problems were detected by FPR in real time. These specific errors would not have been detected with traditional external QC assayed once every 8 hours.

Table 3
Summary of FPR events flagged during a multisite user evaluation of iQM for the GEM Premier 3000

Type of Flag	Number of Samples Flagged	Analytes Affected
Benzalkonium interference	26	Na^+, Ca^{2+}
Unspecified interference	10	Na^+, K^+, Ca^{2+}, Pco_2
Microclots	14	Hematocrit (11), Na^+ (2), Po_2 (1)
Sensor malfunction	3	Glucose, lactate

A total of 10,550 samples were assayed at 4 clinical sites.
Data from Toffaletti JG, McDonnell EH, Ramanathan LV, et al. Validation of a quality assessment system for blood gas and electrolyte testing. Clin Chim Acta 2007;382:65–70.

SUMMARY

Increased emphasis on patient safety in laboratory medicine has placed more demands than ever on detecting error conditions within analytical systems that may lead to incorrect patient results. Minimizing time to detect errors is the key metric of a properly designed QC program. Although most critical care analyzers are capable of self-diagnosis of many failure mechanisms related to hardware, most are not capable of ongoing monitoring of the performance of the entire analytical system. Discrete analysis of QC samples, manually or automatically, detects analytical errors only at the time the QC samples are analyzed, but not with analysis of each patient sample. The move of critical care analysis to POC has resulted in operation of analyzers by personnel untrained in laboratory techniques, in a variety of testing locations. Many operators may not be familiar with the need for a proper QC program. An ongoing, real-time QC program, free of operator intervention, is the most successful QC program at POC.

REFERENCES

1. US hospitals point-of-care study–a multi-client report. Stamford (CT): Enterprise Analysis Corporation; 2011.
2. CLSI. Laboratory quality control based on risk management; approved guideline. CLSI Document EP23-A. Wayne (PA): Clinical and Laboratory Standards Institute; 2011.
3. ISO 14971. Medical devices–application of risk management to medical devices. Geneva (Switzerland): International Organization for Standardization; 2007.
4. Kalra J. Medical errors: impact on clinical laboratories and other critical areas. Clin Biochem 2004;37:1052–62.
5. Plebani M, Carraro P. Mistakes in a stat laboratory: types and frequency. Clin Chem 1997;43:1348–51.
6. Carraro P, Plebani M. Errors in a stat laboratory: types and frequencies 10 years later. Clin Chem 2007;53:1338–42.
7. CLSI. Statistical quality control for quantitative measurement procedures: principles and definitions; approved guideline–3rd edition. CLSI Document C24-A3. Wayne (PA): Clinical and Laboratory Standards Institute; 2006.
8. Westgard JO, Fallon KD, Mansouri S. Validation of iQM active process control technology. Point of Care 2003;2:1–7.
9. Department of Health and Human Services Health Care Financing Administration. Medicare, Medicaid and CLIA programs: regulations implementing the Clinical

Laboratory Improvement Amendments of 1988 (CLIA). Final rule and notice. Fed Regist 1992;57:7002–186.

10. Fallon KD, Ehrmeyer SS, Laessig RH, et al. From quality control and quality assurance to assured quality. Point of Care 2003;2:188–94.

11. Toffaletti JG, McDonnell EH, Ramanathan LV, et al. Validation of a quality assessment system for blood gas and electrolyte testing. Clin Chim Acta 2007;382: 65–70.

Statistical Quality Control Procedures

James O. Westgard, PhD[a,b],*

KEYWORDS

- Statistical quality control • SQC • Sigma-metrics • Control rules
- Analytical run length • CLSI C24A3

KEY POINTS

- The detection capabilities of different control mechanisms are often unknown, except for Statistical QC procedures that can be selected to detect medically important errors.
- The control rules and number of control measurements for SQC procedures should be selected on the basis of the quality required for the intended use of a test and the precision and bias observed for the method.
- SQC should be part of all QC Plans to provide a safety net for detecting medically important errors.

BACKGROUND

The Clinical and Laboratory Standards Institute (CLSI) EP23A[1] recommends a quality control (QC) tool box that includes many different control mechanisms. However, these controls have different performance capabilities, eg, their coverage varies from single-patient samples to single analytical runs to multiple analytical runs. They may target specific components in the analytical system; individual steps in the preanalytical, analytical, or postanalytical processes; the entire analytical process, or the total testing process. In addition, their detection capability may or may not be known.

Running a control does not necessarily mean that medically important errors will be detected. Controls must be carefully designed and their performance should be validated. ISO 15198 provides guidance for "Validation of user quality control procedures by the manufacturer."[2]

> This International Standard is written for manufacturers of in vitro diagnostic (IVD) medical devices as part of their design control and risk management programs. It will also enable manufacturers to provide validated quality control procedures for users in clinical diagnostic laboratories.

[a] Department of Pathology and Laboratory Medicine, University of Wisconsin, Madison, WI 53705, USA; [b] Westgard QC, Inc, 7614 Gray Fox Trail, Madison, WI 53717, USA
* Department of Pathology and Laboratory Medicine, University of Wisconsin, Madison, WI 53705.
E-mail address: james@westgard.com

Clin Lab Med 33 (2013) 111–124
http://dx.doi.org/10.1016/j.cll.2012.10.004
0272-2712/13/$ – see front matter © 2013 Elsevier Inc. All rights reserved.

labmed.theclinics.com

Validation is defined as, "confirmation, through provision of objective evidence, that the requirements for a specific intended use or application have been fulfilled."

The term intended use is consistent with ISO 15189[3] guidance to laboratories (ISO 15198 and ISO 15189 can be confused, but ISO 15198 is guidance for manufacturers and ISO 15189 is guidance for medical laboratories):

5.5 The performance specifications for each procedure used in an examination shall relate to the intended use of that procedure.

5.6.1 The laboratory shall design internal quality control procedures that verify the attainment of the intended quality of results.

A potential shortcoming of the CLSI EP23A guidance is that the recommended risk model neglects detection. It is a 2-factor risk model that considers the probability of occurrence of harm and the severity of harm to prioritize risk and identify appropriate controls to be included in a QC plan. The purpose of that QC plan is to detect failures that would lead to medically important errors, but detection is not part of the risk model.

One way to mitigate this failure is to include a properly designed SQC procedure that is optimized to detect medically important errors. Doing the right SQC right is critical if medical laboratories are to implement proper QC plans. CLSI document C24A3 provide specific guidance for SQC procedures.[4]

DOING THE RIGHT SQC RIGHT

Basic SQC practices are described in general textbooks on laboratory medicine and clinical chemistry,[5] as well as in specific manuals[6] and manufacturers' instructions. The basic practice is to analyze a stable control material again and again to establish the expected range of results. The mean and standard deviation (SD) of the control results are calculated and control charts or control rules are established. The standard graphical presentation is the Levey-Jennings control chart, which presents the control result on the y-axis versus time on the x-axis. Control limits are established as the mean plus and minus a certain multiple of the SD, commonly the mean $\pm$ 2 SD or the mean $\pm$ 3 SD, which may also identified as a 1_{2s} or 1_{3s} control rule, respectively. As an alternative, multiple control rules may be applied simultaneously in what is known as multirule SQC[7] (sometimes called Westgard rules). See **Box 1** for definitions of commonly used control rules.

SQC is a well-established practice in medical laboratories; nonetheless, SQC is sometimes problematic because the wrong control rules are often used. For example, the use of 2 SD control limits on Levey-Jennings control charts leads to approximately 10% false rejections when 2 levels of control are being analyzed, which is the minimum or default requirement in the US Clinical Laboratory Improvement Amendments (CLIA) regulations. Because of false rejections, many laboratories respond to an out-of-control situation by just repeating controls, again and again, until they are in. In effect, laboratories often do the wrong QC wrong, and analysts and operators get frustrated by the ongoing control problems. The remedy is to first select the right SQC procedure, then to implement SQC right.

SQC Process

Fig. 1 provides an overview of the steps in the SQC process in a medical laboratory and also identifies who is responsible for each of these steps. SQC is a shared responsibility between laboratory managers and analysts. In large laboratories, there may be quality specialists who exercise the management responsibilities, but all analysts

---

Box 1
Control rule definitions

- 1_{2s} refers to the control rule commonly used with a Levey-Jennings chart, in which control limits are set as the mean ± 2 SD. This rule is sometimes used as a rejection rule, in which case there often are problems with false rejections (5% for N = 1, 10% for N = 2). In multirule SQC procedures, this rule is used as a warning rule to trigger careful inspection of the control data by other rejection rules.

- 1_{3s}: reject when 1 control measurement exceeds the mean ± 3 SD

- $1_{2.5s}$: reject when 1 control measurement exceeds the mean ± 2.5 SD control limits.

- 2_{2s}: reject when 2 consecutive control measurements exceed the same mean + 2 SD control limit or the same mean − 2 SD control limit.

- $2of3_{2s}$: reject when 2 out of 3 control measurements exceed the same mean + 2 SD or mean − 2 SD control limit.

- R_{4s}: reject when 1 control measurement in a group exceeds the mean + 2 SD control limit and another exceeds the mean − 2 SD control limit. Note: this rule is best applied within a single rule.

- 3_{1s}: reject when 3 consecutive control measurements exceed the same mean + 1 SD or the same mean − 1 SD control limit.

- 4_{1s}: reject when 4 consecutive control measurements exceed the same mean + 1 SD or the same mean − 1 SD control limit.

- 6x: reject when 6 consecutive control measurements are on 1 side of the mean.

- 8x: reject when 8 consecutive control measurements are on 1 side of the mean.

- 10x: reject when 10 consecutive control measurements are on 1 side of the mean.

Data from Westgard JO. Basic QC practices. 3rd edition. Madison (WI): Westgard QC; 2011.

---

should be involved so that QC is part of their responsibilities to the physician customers and patient consumers.

Doing the right SQC means selecting the right control rules and the right number of control measurements for the quality required for the test and the precision and bias

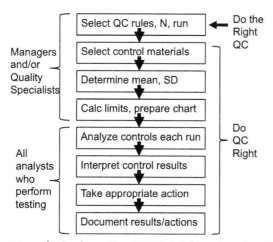

Fig. 1. Laboratory process for implementing SQC. N, total number of control measurements; SD, standard deviation.

observed for the method. Doing SQC right depends on proper implementation of the selected SQC procedure, which involves selecting control materials, determining the mean and SD, calculating control limits and preparing a control chart, or selecting the right control rules in a computerized QC charting program. These activities are the responsibility of laboratory managers or quality specialists.

Doing SQC right also involves the daily activities for analysis of controls in each analytical run, interpretation of the control results, followed by appropriate actions to release test results or undertake corrective actions, concluding with documentation of those actions. These activities are the responsibility of all analysts who perform testing.

DOING THE RIGHT SQC

ISO 15198 recommends SQC as a generally applicable control procedure:

> For existing IVD medical devices, conventional statistical quality control procedures (eg, as described in CLSI C24) are considered adequate unless evidence from risk-monitoring activities indicates [other] quality control procedures are essential for maintaining risk at an acceptable level. In such cases, the quality control procedures shall be validated .... NOTE: Demonstration that a statistical quality control procedure will detect results that exceed predetermined limits does not require induction of actual failure modes. Validation may be based on statistical evaluation of the simulated effects of imprecision and/or bias on actual performance data obtained in routine operating mode.

There are 2 important points here: (1) SQC procedures can be readily validated based on existing information on their rejection characteristics, as determined from simulation studies documented in the clinical chemistry literature (Refs.[8–14] cited in ISO 15198). (2) Validation of other control procedures will likely require induction of failure modes to determine whether the QC procedures will detect medically important errors. Manufacturers can do this in the validation of new systems, but laboratories will find it difficult to induce specific failures to validate detection of individual controls. SQC is essential because it is an independent control that can be designed to provide the necessary error detection.

SQC Planning Process

CLSI C24A3 describes how to select a valid SQC procedure by using the planning process shown in **Fig. 2**. The first step is to define the quality specification for the test. Quality specification here means the quality goal for the intended use. Next, the laboratory selects appropriate control materials and determines method performance. The laboratory may already have this information available from method validation studies or from ongoing SQC data. What is important is to combine the defined quality goal and the observed method performance to calculate a sigma-metric:

Sigma = (%TEa − %Bias)/%CV

where *TEa* is the allowable total error, *Bias* is the observed inaccuracy of the method, and *CV* is the observed imprecision of the method. All terms must be in the same units, either concentration or percent. Many of the CLIA criteria for acceptable performance in proficiency testing are stated as a percentage of target value, so it is generally convenient to consider all terms as percentages.

The next step is to identify candidate SQC strategies. In CLSI C24A3, a QC strategy is defined as "the number of control materials, the number of measurements to be made on those materials, the location of those control materials in an analytical run,

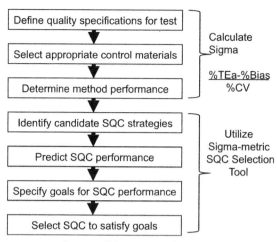

Fig. 2. Planning process to select a valid SQC procedure. CV, coefficient of variation.

and the statistical quality control rules applied." Candidate SQC strategies should reflect the choice of 2 or 3 different levels of controls, location of the controls for batch operation or for continuous reporting of test results, the control rules for interpreting the control measurements, and the total number of control measurements that are needed.

To predict SQC performance, a common approach is to use available power curves that describe the probability for rejection versus the size of analytical errors. For a specific application, 2 characteristics are important: the probability for false rejection (P_{fr}) and the probability for error detection (P_{ed}). The goal for P_{ed} is commonly set as greater than or equal to 0.90 or 90% detection of medically important systematic errors. The goal for P_{fr} is commonly set as less than or equal to 0.05 or 5% false rejections.

Sigma-metric QC Selection Tool

The power curves for commonly used SQC procedures are shown in **Fig. 3**. The probability for rejection is plotted on the y-axis versus the size of systematic error on the lower x-axis, or the value of the sigma-metric on the upper x-axis. The different curves correspond, top to bottom, with the list of SQC procedures shown top to bottom in the key at the right. The key identifies the control rules and the total number of control measurements. Note that this particular tool is to be used for 2 levels of controls because all values of N are all multiples of 2. The goal for error detection is shown by the dashed horizontal line that intersects the y-axis at 0.90. The goal for false rejection is indicated as 0.05 on the y-axis. The dotted vertical lines represent different sizes of medically important errors (bottom x-scale) or different sigma-metrics (top x-scale). If methods achieve world-class quality (ie, 6 sigma performance, which is slightly off the scale to the right), all of the power curves would plateau above 0.90 and all of these SQC procedures would achieve the desired error detection. The best choice is to use the SQC procedure with the simplest rules, lowest N, and lowest probability for false rejection, such as the $1_{3.5s}$ single rule with N = 2 and a false rejection of 0.00.

Example for sigma = 5.0

Fig. 4 shows a test in which TEa is 10%, bias is 0%, CV is 2%, and sigma is 5.0 [(10−0)/2]. To select an appropriate SQC procedure, identify the sigma-metric on the scale at the top, drop a vertical line, observe where that line intersects the power curves, then read the probabilities for error detection on the y-axis. Note that the

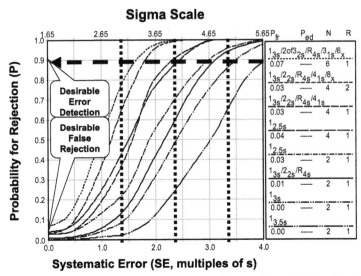

Fig. 3. Sigma-metric QC selection tool for 2 levels of controls. Probability for rejection is shown on y-axis vs size of systematic error on bottom scale of x-axis and sigma-metric on top scale of x-axis. Power curves top to bottom represent the different QC procedures top to bottom in the key at the right. Desirable error detection is shown by dashed line at top. False rejection is indicated by y-intercept of a power curve. Dotted vertical lines represent sigma values of 3, 4, and 5. Control rules defined in **Box 1**; N, total number of control measurements; P_{ed}, probability of error detection; P_{fr}, probability of false rejection; R, number of runs over which control rules are applied; s, standard deviation.

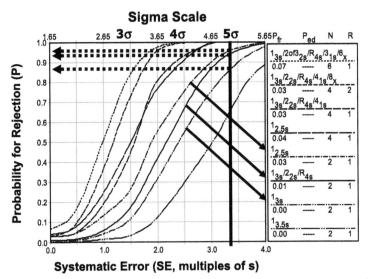

Fig. 4. Example application for 5-sigma testing process. Dashed lines at top illustrate expected error detection for 3 QC procedures that are identified in the key at the right by the solid lines with arrows. Control rules defined in **Box 1**; N, total number of control measurements; Ped, probability of error detection; Pfr, probability of false rejection; R, number of runs over which control rules are applied; s, standard deviation.

4 power curves on the left all achieve 100% error detection, but require 4 to 6 control measurements per run. The curves of most interest are the next 3, which require fewer control measurements and have probabilities for error detection of about 0.96, 0.94, and 0.87. These 3 control procedures can be identified in the key at the right as $1_{2.5s}$ with N = 2, $1_{3s}/2_{2s}/R_{4s}$ with N = 2, and 1_{3s} with N = 2. Their probabilities for false rejection are determined from the y-intercepts of the power curves and are given in the key as 0.03, 0.01, and 0.00, respectively. Considering the goals for SQC performance, all 3 satisfy the goal for P_{fr} less than or equal to 0.05 and 2 of those also satisfy the goal for P_{ed} greater than or equal to 0.90. Therefore, the best choices are to implement $1_{2.5s}$ with N = 2 or $1_{3s}/2_{2s}/R_{4s}$ with N = 2. However, in some situations, it may be appropriate to implement 1_{3s} with N = 2 because that is a simpler SQC procedure, particularly for manual preparation of Levey-Jennings charts with control limits set as the mean ± 3 SD.

Example for sigma = 4.0
A second example is shown in **Fig. 5**, in which TEa is 10%, bias is 2%, CV is 2%, and sigma is 4.0 [(10−2)/2]. The 2 SQC procedures of most interest here are the $1_{3s}/2_{2s}/R_{4s}/4_{1s}$ multirule with N = 4 or the $1_{2.5s}$ single rule with N = 4. The 2 are close in performance, with P_{fr} of 0.03 and 0.04, respectively, and P_{ed} of 0.91 and 0.88, respectively. In principle, the multirule procedure is a better choice, but the performance is so close that either would be appropriate. The decision between the two may be based on practical issues in implementing the rules. Some SQC software may not support multirules, and other software may not support use of 2.5 SD control limits. Manual applications may be simpler if only a single rule is used. In contrast, manual implementation of 2.5 SD control limits may create some confusion because common practices are mainly to use 2 SD or 3 SD control limits. In that case, it may be easier to implement the multirule procedure, even for manual applications.

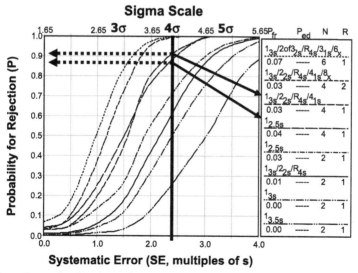

Fig. 5. Example application for 4-sigma testing process. Dashed lines at top illustrate expected error detection for 2 QC procedures that are identified in the key at the right by the solid lines with arrows. Control rules defined in **Box 1**; N, total number of control measurements; P_{ed}, probability of error detection; P_{fr}, probability of false rejection; R, number of runs over which control rules are applied; s, standard deviation.

Example for sigma = 3.3

Fig. 6 shows an application in which TEa is 10%, bias is 0.0%, CV is 3.0%, and sigma is 3.3 [(10−0)/3]. The appropriate SQC procedures are both multirule procedures, one with 6 control measurements per run and the other with 4 control measurements per run, but with inspection of controls over 2 runs (that is the meaning of R = 2 in the key). The best choice is the N = 6 procedure because it provides the necessary error detection in a single run. The difficulty with that procedure is that it is expensive to analyze that many controls. The alternative is to analyze 4 controls and then use an 8x rule to look back at control data from the previous rule to obtain the necessary 8 measurements for that rule. Neither is ideal, but the problem is that the method performs so poorly that it is difficult and costly for a laboratory to do enough SQC to provide the necessary error detection.

Summary Guidance for Selecting the Right SQC

Based on these examples, there are some simple rules to provide guidance for selecting SQC procedures:

- For methods in which sigma achieves the goal of world-class quality (ie, 6 sigma), any SQC will do, but ensure that 2 SD limits are not being used because there is no need to tolerate a high level of false rejections. Use 3 or even 3.5 SD limits to minimize false rejections and a maximum of 2 or 3 control measurements.
- For methods in which sigma is greater than or equal to 5.0, 2 control measurements and single control rules such as $1_{2.5s}$ or even 1_{3s} provide the necessary error detection with 2 or 3 control measurements.
- For methods in which sigma is between 4.9 and 3.6, more controls are needed. Doubling the number of controls to a total of 4 to 6 is a good practice.

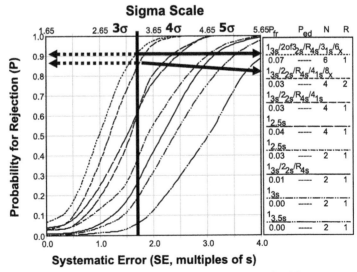

Fig. 6. Example application for 3.3-sigma testing process. Dashed lines at top illustrate expected error detection for 2 QC procedure that are identified in the key at the right by solid lines with arrows. Control rules defined in **Box 1**; N, total number of control measurements; P_{ed}, probability of error detection; P_{fr}, probability of false rejection; R, number of runs over which control rules are applied; s, standard deviation.

- For methods in which sigma is 4.0 or less, multirule SQC procedures should be implemented to maximize error detection.
- For methods in which sigma is less than or equal to 3.4, a laboratory should perform the maximum SQC that it can afford, but it should also implement other control mechanisms to prevent errors from occurring and to improve detection of errors.
- For methods in which sigma is between 3.5 and 4.9, careful application of the sigma-metric QC selection tool is advised to provide the optimal control rules and number of control measurements.

DOING SQC RIGHT

As shown in **Fig. 1**, doing SQC right involves selecting control materials, determining their mean and SD, calculating control limits and implementing control rules with graphical control charts or SQC software, analyzing controls each run (as defined by the standard operating procedure [SOP] for the test), interpreting control results, taking appropriate action, and documenting the results and actions. Setting up the SQC procedure and defining the SOP are management responsibilities. The remaining steps are the responsibility of all the analysts in the laboratory.

Selection of Control Materials

Control materials should behave like patient samples. Laboratories used to prepare their own patient pools for use as controls, but they now purchase control materials from manufacturers who specialize in their production. The matrix of those commercial control materials should be the same as the patient samples, but there are practical limitations caused by the additives and processing that are necessary to ensure long-term stability. For example, lyophilized materials are different from fresh liquid patient samples. Likewise, liquid control materials contain additives that make them different from fresh patient samples. These differences may lead to matrix effects, whereby different methods obtain different test results on the same control material. That is not necessarily a serious problem when the control materials are used for an individual method and the mean and SD are established from repetitive testing with that method. However, commutability is particularly an issue for materials that have assigned values that are expected to be correct for different methods and analytical systems, or when such materials are used in proficiency testing and external quality-assessment programs to evaluate laboratory performance.

Stability is an important issue, both long term and from vial to vial. Control materials should be stable for a year or longer to minimize difficulties of changing from one lot number to another. Vial-to-vial variability should be minimal so that the observed variability reflects primarily the analytical variability of the method. Liquid materials have an advantage for minimizing vial-to-vial variability, but may introduce problems with viscosity. Control materials generally achieve the desired stability for much of the testing in clinical chemistry, but they have limited stability in other areas, such as hematology cell counts.

Target values (ie, the mean concentrations for different analytes) should be close to medically important decision levels. However, multianalyte controls that have 20 or 40 or more analytes are not likely to meet the target values for all of those analytes. For critical tests, such as hemoglobin A1c, special controls may be needed that are intended primarily for those tests. General practice in clinical chemistry is to analyze 2 levels of controls, whereas 3 levels of controls are often analyzed for blood gas measurements, immunoassays, and hematology testing.

Determination of Mean and SD

Although both assayed and unassayed control materials are available, it is generally recommended that a laboratory establish its own mean and SD from a minimum of 20 measurements over a period of 20 days, each from a different vial of control material. Longer term estimates of means and SDs may be based on cumulative data obtained over several months to account for the effects of changes in reagent lots, calibrations, operator variability, and environmental conditions. Cumulative control limits may be based on 3 to 6 months of control data to provide reliable estimates of process performance.

Calculation of Control Limits

Control limits should be calculated from the mean and SD determined in the laboratory by the particular method operating under stable conditions. The use of bottle values or values from assayed materials is not recommended, except as a stopgap when introducing a new lot of materials that has not been analyzed in parallel with the old lot. Likewise, the use of group values for the mean and SD from peer-comparison programs is not recommended. Such practices have been used in laboratories to widen control limits and reduce the false rejections resulting from 2 SD control limits. The preferred practice is to select the right SQC rules and avoid the use of 2 SD control limits, followed by use of the mean and SD determined in the laboratory to calculate the control limits.

SQC software may allow use of assayed values, user assigned values, monthly values, moving interval values, or cumulative values. Management personnel are responsible for setting up the control limits so that the selected control rules provide the desired performance, which may require a detailed understanding of the working of the SQC software to implement control limits that reflect the laboratory's own performance limits.

Management personnel are also responsible for establishing the SQC strategy as part of the SOP for the test and method. This process includes specifying the control rules (which includes how the control limits are calculated), the number of levels of control materials, the number of measurements on each level of control material, the location of the controls in an analytical run, and the frequency of analysis of the controls. Thereafter, individual analysts or operators are responsible for following the specified SQC strategy.

Analysis of Controls in Each Run

The issue here is how often controls should be analyzed, which is sometimes discussed as frequency of controls and also as run length. Here is the guidance from CLSI C24A3:

> For purposes of quality control, the laboratory must consider the stability of the analytical testing process, its susceptibility to problems that may occur, and the risk associated with an undetected error.

> An analytical run is an interval (ie, a period of time or series of measurements) within which the accuracy and precision of the measuring system is expected to be stable; between which events may occur causing the measurement process to be more susceptible (ie, greater risk) to errors that are important to detect.

The important ideas are stability, susceptibility, and risk; an interval, period of time, or number of patient specimens for which the measurement system is expected to be stable, and between which events may occur. Events are the key to making practical sense of this guidance. Consider frequency of QC to be event driven, as discussed by Parvin.[14] There are expected events, such as the daily setup of an analyzer, a change of reagents, a new lot of calibrators, replacement of an instrument component, preventive maintenance, and possibly the change of analysts or operators. There are also unexpected events, such as reagent deterioration, instrument drift, failure of an instrument component, and change of environmental conditions such as temperature or humidity. Controls are needed to evaluate the effects of these events. For expected events, the controls can be scheduled for the event. For unexpected events, controls must be analyzed periodically to ensure that these changes do not cause medically important errors.

Risk analysis should help laboratories identify events or failure modes. Likewise, risk analysis should help prioritize their importance and how they can be detected. The QC plan should then schedule controls for the times of known events and also schedule controls to provide periodic monitoring of unexpected events. As a general SQC strategy, regulatory requirements set a minimum frequency of 2 levels of controls per day. To this minimum, the laboratory should add controls for known events to assess the significance of changes in the testing process, plus additional periodic controls to monitor for unexpected events during routine production.

Dooley[15] pointed out that the frequency of QC should also consider the immediacy of use of the test and the physician's test repeat cycle. If a wrong test result is reported, it may be expected that the physician will reorder the test to confirm the result. The laboratory should have performed SQC in the interval between the original test and the repeat test so that any problem would have been detected and corrected. Controls should therefore be analyzed more often for tests provided to an intensive care unit than for tests for outpatient service. According to Dooley[15]:

With patient safety in mind, the rationale for the frequency of QC becomes quite simple, in contrast with other approaches being developed and applied by manufacturers for assessing and mitigating the risk of failure of their analytic systems and by laboratories for mitigating the remaining 'residual risks' for those changes that occur under routine laboratory operations. In a sense, this is risk management too, but made simple by focusing on the physician and patient, not the manufacturer and instrument. The important point is that this approach would ensure that the physician continues to have the opportunity to reduce the risk that an erroneous laboratory result poses for the patient.

Interpretation of Control Results

The laboratory's SOPs should define the SQC procedure and provide directions for interpreting control results. Graphical displays of control data on Levey-Jennings charts are useful for a visual assessment, but it is necessary to define specific control rules to ensure systematic and uniform interpretation by all analysts and operators. Single-rule SQC procedures are preferred for manual applications and low-volume testing sites, but the methodology used in these sites may require a greater number of control measurements and possibly multirule interpretation of the control results. Use of 2.5 SD control limits, or a $1_{2.5s}$ control rule, provides about the same error detection as a multirule procedure with the same N, but, as N increases, the false rejections are greater for the $1_{2.5s}$ control rule.

Appropriate Action

The laboratory's SOPs should also describe the appropriate actions that are to be taken when control results are in control or out of control. CLSI C24A3 advises that the common practice of repeating control measurements should be avoided, which emphasizes the importance of selecting the right SQC procedure to minimize false rejections and maximize error detection. Instead of repeating controls, laboratories should investigate the problem, identify its cause, and take corrective actions. The performance of the testing process then should be reevaluated, any questionable patient test results should be examined, and, if necessary, the tests should be repeated.

Documentation of Results and Actions

Control results and the corresponding actions should be documented to provide an accurate history of process performance. Given the importance of events, all changes that are made to the testing process must also be documented. Such changes should be reviewed whenever control problems occur. Those changes that make the process susceptible to errors should be identified for preventive actions and should be monitored by event-driven SQC. The control record of a testing process is often the most valuable information for improving the QC Plan.

ASSESSMENT OF SQC DESIGN AND PRACTICES IN YOUR LABORATORY

The worksheet shown in **Fig. 7** should be helpful for auditing the SQC practices in your laboratory. The top half focuses on method performance (TEa, precision, bias) and the calculation of sigma-metrics, which can then be used to assess the right SQC rules and right number of control measurements, plus provide guidance for a sigma TQC strategy that can prioritize the need for risk analysis and different QC tools.

The bottom half of the worksheet concerns your present SQC practices, beginning with the control chart parameters and the current control rules and number of control measurements (ie, your current SQC design). The remaining parts of the worksheet relate to the SQC practices in your laboratory. All these factors influence the effectiveness of your SQC procedures in routine operation.

Do not be surprised if the SQC practices differ from what is written in the laboratory's SOPs. Some of the common things that may be wrong with current SQC practices are as follows:

- Wrong QC design, particularly the use of 2 SD control limits, which cause a high probability for false rejections
- Misuse of bottle values, assigned values, and peer-group data for means and SDs for calculation of control limits
- Controls analyzed in advance with no monitoring of the length of the analytical run
- Frequency of control testing set to comply with minimum regulatory requirements, rather than to ensure the quality needed for patient care
- Wrong response to out-of-control signals: repeat controls until the results are in control
- Lack of corrective and preventive actions to improve quality of testing

Performing an audit of the SQC practices in your laboratory may be the best first step for improving QC.

WHAT IS THE POINT?

An SQC procedure will not perform as needed for patient care unless the laboratory establishes the right control rules, right number of control measurements, and the right run length or right frequency of SQC in the SOP.

An SQC procedure will not perform as expected for laboratory operation unless the right mean and SD are used, the right control limits are calculated, the right interpretation is made of the control data, and the right actions are taken.

Laboratory Assessment of SQC Design and SQC Practices Worksheet
Laboratory Section   _Analyst_   _Date_

Method Performance Characteristics and SQC Design

Test (Units)				
Method (Analyzer)				
Medical Decision Levels		LOW Xc	MID Xc	High Xc
	Concentrations			
CLIA Quality Criterion	%TEa			
Precision (Replication or QC Data)	SD			
	Mean			
	%CV			
Bias (Comparison, PT, Peer Data)	Calculated Bias			
	%Bias			
Sigma-Metric	(%TEa)/%CV			
	(%TEa - %Bias)/%CV			
SQC from Sigma tool, Control Rules				
Total Number Measurements, N				
Sigma QC Strategy				

Laboratory SQC Practices

Number of Control Materials		Low	Mid	High
Control Chart Parameters	SD			
	Mean			
	%CV			
Control Rules Used				
Total N Used				
Mode of Operation	Continuous or Batch or Unit Use			
Number of Operators				
Number Patient Samples/Run or Day				
Service Priority/Turnaround Time				
Location of Controls				
Frequency of Controls				
Events requiring QC				
Response to 1st Out-of-Control				
Response to 2nd Out-of-Control				
Practice for Calc Initial Control Limits				
Practice for Updating Control Limits				
Occurrence, Frequency of problems	Low <2% or Mod 2%-10% or High >10%			

Fig. 7. Worksheet for auditing laboratory SQC applications. CV, coefficient of variation; High Xc, high decision level concentration; LOW Xc, low decision level concentration; MID Xc, mid decision level concentration; N, total number of control measurements; SD, standard deviation; TEa, allowable Total Error.

Doing the right SQC right is not easy, but it is essential in any QC plan to provide a safety net for detecting medically important errors.

REFERENCES

1. CLSI EP23A. Laboratory quality control based on risk management. Wayne (PA): Clinical and Laboratory Standards Institute; 2011.

2. ISO 15198. Clinical laboratory medicine – in vitro diagnostic medical devices – validation of user quality control procedures by the manufacturer. Geneva (Switzerland): ISO; 2004.
3. ISO 15189. Medical laboratories – particular requirements for quality and competence. Geneva (Switzerland): ISO; 2007.
4. CLSI C24A3. Statistical quality control for quantitative measurement procedures. Wayne (PA): Clinical and Laboratory Standards Institute; 2006.
5. Klee GG, Westgard JO. Quality management. Chapter 8. In: Burtis CA, Ashwood ER, Bruns DE, editors. Tietz textbook of clinical chemistry and molecular diagnostics. St Louis (MO): Elsevier Saunders; 2012. p. 163–203.
6. Westgard JO. Basic QC practices. 3rd edition. Madison (WI): Westgard QC; 2011.
7. Westgard JO, Barry PL, Hunt MR, et al. A multi-rule Shewhart chart for quality control in clinical chemistry. Clin Chem 1981;27:493–501.
8. Westgard JO, Barry PL. Cost effective quality control: managing the quality and productivity of analytical processes. Washington, DC: AACC Press; 1986.
9. Westgard JO, Stein B. An automatic process for selecting statistical QC procedures to assure clinical and analytical quality requirements. Clin Chem 1997; 43:400–3.
10. Parvin CA. Quality-control (QC) performance measures and the QC planning process. Clin Chem 1997;43:602–7.
11. Westgard JO. Basic planning for quality. Madison (WI): Westgard QC; 2000.
12. Brooks ZC. Performance-driven quality control. Washington (DC): AACC Press; 2001.
13. Westgard JO. Six sigma quality design and control. Madison (WI): Westgard QC; 2001.
14. Parvin CA. Assessing the impact of the frequency of quality control testing on the quality of reported patient results. Clin Chem 2008;54:2049–54.
15. Dooley KC. Frequency of QC: a patient safety perspective. Available at: www.westgard.com/guest35.htm. Accessed September 15, 2012.

Accuracy Controls
Assessing Trueness (Bias)

David Armbruster, PhD, DABCC, FACB

KEYWORDS

- Accuracy controls • Bias • Trueness • Allowable total error (TEa)
- Statistical quality control (SQC) • Systematic error (SE) • Random error (RE)

KEY POINTS

- Precision controls monitor assay random error (reproducibility) and accuracy controls assess total error, both random error and systematic error.
- Trueness (bias) of an assay represents systematic error.
- An accuracy control should be metrologically traceable, ideally with a target value determined by use of a reference material or a reference method.
- An accuracy control should be commutable and its analytical response to a reference method and a routine field method should be equivalent to that of a patient sample.
- Accuracy controls should be prepared by the providers of reference materials and manufactured in the same fashion as a calibrator.

THE GOAL OF QUALITY CONTROL

"Since the output of clinical chemistry laboratories is either expressed in numbers or is opinion based on numerical information, it is important that all concerned with its use should know the reliability of the data involved. In retrospect, it is surprising that the necessity for this did not appear to a science-based profession before the beginning of the last decade. Since then, quality control has followed a predictable course of evolution: first covering local needs, then national, and now international. It is at present changing in nature from the control of precision to the control of accuracy."[1] This observation is very appropriate for the twenty-first century, but it was actually written by Mitchell[1] in 1975. Similar sentiments were expressed even earlier (1971) by Caraway,[2] who wrote "The expression 'accurate enough for clinical purposes' has an inference demeaning to the medical profession, and poor implications as to the adequacy of our work as clinical chemists. Experience shows that improved accuracy and specificity lead to better discrimination in diagnosis and treatment ..." and "A reported value whose accuracy is entirely unknown is worthless." The importance of

Disclosure: David Armbruster is an employee of Abbott Diagnostics.
Global Scientific Affairs, Abbott Diagnostics, Department 09AA/Building CP1-5, 100 Abbott Park Road, Abbott Park, IL 60064-6096, USA
E-mail address: David.Armbruster@abbott.com

Clin Lab Med 33 (2013) 125–137
http://dx.doi.org/10.1016/j.cll.2012.10.002
0272-2712/13/$ – see front matter © 2013 Elsevier Inc. All rights reserved.

assessing accuracy of patient test results has long been recognized in the clinical laboratory field, yet the typical approach to quality controls consists of monitoring precision, in the form of standard deviation (SD) or coefficient of variation (%CV), and not trueness/bias in the form of the closeness of a test result to a predetermined target value. If accuracy is the goal, then quality control samples need to assess both precision and trueness of an analytical procedure. A risk management–based approach to ensure test quality and conduct quality control obviously must include accuracy.

The reality is that test results obtained from a clinical laboratory in one region or country may not be comparable with results generated for the same patient sample tested by another laboratory.[3] This is because the assays for many analytes are not standardized. Without standardization, the differences between results from 2 or more laboratories may not be clinically interpretable; that is, they are inconsistent and suggest different medical conditions. This is a very real problem because standardized clinical practice guidelines, whose use is encouraged by evidence-based laboratory medicine (EBLM), in many cases dictate action or treatment when a test result is either greater or less than a given medical decision level (MDL). These MDLs are assumed to be independent of the methodology used to obtain the results. For example, further action may be taken when a cholesterol value is greater than 5.2 mmol/L (200 mg/dL) or a prostate specific antigen (PSA) result exceeds 4.0 µg/L (4.0 ng/mL), no matter what method is used to generate the value. In the case of cholesterol, the typical field methods are sufficiently standardized to ensure that reliable decisions are made. For PSA, however, that is not the case.[4] Accuracy controls allow test results to be assessed against an absolute, as opposed to a relative, measure of trueness and can ensure that test results are suitably reliable for clinical purposes.

Clinical guidelines often recommend CVs for analytical imprecision without appropriate specifications (eg, within day, total) and that are not based on biologic variation and medical use, causing a major problem in establishing quality requirements. The assumption is that reproducibility of an assay is sufficient to produce an accurate result. Even when precision in terms of %CV is specified, it is not sufficient to guarantee the allowable limit for trueness/bias is not exceeded because precision alone cannot act as a surrogate for accuracy. There is a distinction between clinical accuracy (ie, whether a test successfully distinguishes between health and disease or different stages of a disease), and analytical accuracy (ie, how close the result of a field method is to the true value as determined by a reference method target value).[5] It is the responsibility of the clinical laboratory to provide analytically accurate patient test results.

The goal of clinical laboratories is to produce patient test results that are comparable to the point of being interchangeable (ie, essentially equivalent), and that are also accurate. Rosenbaum,[6] in 1985, demonstrated that agreement between reference method target values for some analytes; for example, Na and K by flame atomic emission spectroscopy and Ca by isotope dilution-mass spectrometry, and all method means for field methods was good when using human serum pools as samples. Bias with glucose, however, was significant (+5%) and was variable for cholesterol. Quality controls should assess and monitor accuracy of clinical laboratory tests by reflecting both precision and bias, and not repeatability alone.

DEFINITIONS

To understand the distinction between precision and accuracy controls, it is useful to review some standard definitions from the *International Vocabulary of Metrology*.[7] Precision is defined as closeness of agreement between independent test result obtained under stipulated conditions, or repeatability (reproducibility), or random error (RE). RE is the component of measurement error that in replicate measurements varies in an unpredictable manner. Measurement precision is determined by replicate measurements on the same sample under specified conditions and is usually expressed by SD or CV or %CV. Statistical quality control (SQC) typically is considered to reflect precision.

Bias is the amount by which a result varies from the correct result. Trueness is the closeness of agreement between the average value from replicate test results and the target value determined by a reference method. Measurement trueness is inversely related to systematic measurement error, but is not related to random measurement error. For sake of simplicity, bias and trueness can be considered to be interchangeable. Systematic error (SE) is the component of measurement error that in replicate measurements remains constant or varies in a predictable manner. Trueness/bias is an estimate of SE. A fundamental principle is that "trueness" can be defined only through "traceability."[8]

Accuracy is defined as the closeness of agreement between the result of a measurement and a true value of the measurand, when the true value is a value consistent with the definition of a given quantity, ideally a measurement with no errors, random or systematic. Accuracy reflects the ability of the measurement procedure to give the correct result. It is significant to note that, according to metrology, the article "a" is used with true value instead of the article "the" because there can be many "true values" consistent with the definition of a given quantity. Hence, there is no certainty that the mean of a precision control is the "true value." Accuracy is the combination of trueness (bias) and precision, so the smaller the bias and the better the precision, the more accurate the measurement. Clearly, neither trueness nor precision alone can be equated with or define accuracy.

A measurand is the particular quantity subject to measurement, which for practical purposes in the clinical laboratory can be considered an analyte in a specific matrix (eg, glucose in serum, or plasma, or cerebrospinal fluid, or urine). Measurand differs from "analyte," or the name of a substance or compound, although the terms are sometimes used interchangeably. This usage is erroneous because analyte does not refer to quantities.

Total error allowable (TEa) is the sum of random RE (precision) and SE (trueness/bias). Control measurements inherently contain both RE and SE. The RE reflects the spread of values attributable to imprecision, and the SE shifts the mean of the control in one direction or the other from the "true value." For any analysis, the goal is to ensure the observed total error (TE) does not exceed the TEa (TE < TEa).

The ideal role of SQC is ideally to detect random and systematic errors and to ensure that TEa is not exceeded. Because TEa depends on precision and bias, some measurands require more or less rigorous control rules.

As Caraway noted, "Intuitively, we all know what we mean by accuracy. A given sample of serum, for example, must contain one and only one *true* concentration of calcium. Accuracy is closeness to the 'true' value. We admit that we do not know the true value of substances in biologic material since different methods frequently give different results."[2]

Three more definitions are of interest when discussing accuracy controls. Verification is confirmation, through the provision of objective evidence, that specified requirements have been fulfilled. This means that an assay has been designed and manufactured to meet predetermined performance specifications (ie, that the assay was "built right"). Validation, in contrast, is confirmation, through objective evidence, that the requirements for a specific intended use or application have been fulfilled (ie, that an assay is "fit for purpose" and that the "right assay" was built for clinical purposes). The point is that an assay must not only meet manufacturing design specifications but must also be clinically useful. A precision control can be used to determine if an assay meets precision requirements, but an accuracy control is needed to confirm that an assay conforms to accuracy specifications. Commutability of a reference material, such as an accuracy control, is demonstrated by the closeness of agreement between the relation among the measurement results for a stated quantity in this material, obtained according to 2 given measurement procedures, and the relation obtained among the measurement results for other specified materials. This definition is obscure, which is not unusual in metrology, and means that a control demonstrates an analytical response equivalent to that of a routine patient sample when tested using a reference method and one or more field methods. Or in other words, a control does not exhibit what is commonly called matrix effects.

TE AND TEA

A quality-control sample should provide evidence that an assay under typical conditions provides results that do not exceed the TEa target value. As Eisenhart[9] explains "The *bias*, or *systematic error*, of a measurement process is the magnitude and direction of its tendency to measure something other than what was intended; its *precision* refers to the typical closeness together of successive independent measurements of a single magnitude generated by repeated applications of the process under specified conditions; and its *accuracy* is determined by the closeness to the true value characteristic of such measurements." The TEa target dictates the acceptable precision and accuracy of a method.[10] Unfortunately, most clinical laboratories still do not use objective quality goals when choosing and implementing test procedures. In addition, EBLM guidelines often do not provide specifications for precision, accuracy, and quality control. In general, laboratory error must be less than the biologic variation of an analyte to determine if a difference between 2 sequential results signifies a clinically significant change in a patient, but it is uncertain how much less than the observed biologic variability the error must be. The inherent quality of assays is generally assumed but often is not objectively proven, as it could be by use of accuracy controls that provide an estimate of the total error of a measurement.

The International Federation of Clinical Chemistry (IFCC) defines accuracy as the "agreement between the best estimate of a quantity and its true value."[11] The term inaccuracy, often used to describe the disagreement between the measured value and the true value, is defined by the IFCC as the "numerical difference between the mean of a set of replicate measurements and the true value." These IFCC definitions imply a "systematic error concept of accuracy" (ie, only systematic differences are included when the mean of a group of replicates is used to estimate inaccuracy). Westgard prefers to consider an "overall error concept of accuracy," that is, inaccuracy is the numerical difference between a test result and the true value, and may include both random and systematic error.[10] Ideally, then, an accuracy control sample should be used to assess total error, including both precision and trueness/bias.

As noted by Büttner,[12] "Fundamentally, a measurement without error is not possible. Since the work of Carl Friedrich Gauss, we make a distinction between the constant errors, also referred to as systematic errors, and the variable random errors. The definition of errors is based on the mental assumption that a 'true value' of the measured quantity exists. The 'true value' is a theoretical concept; it is not possible experimentally to exactly determine this true value by measurement. It is therefore expedient to define operationally a 'conventional true value' for practical purposes." He continues to explain that determination of trueness/bias is more difficult than precision, because it has to be estimated using an accepted "true value," presumably assigned by a reference method, whereas the random errors can be estimated by a large number of replicate measurements. It is not surprising that typical quality controls are precision controls and why accuracy controls are rare. But given that accuracy consists of both trueness/bias and precision, systematic error must be addressed and requires accuracy controls.

Systematic errors typically are the cause of the observed deviations between methods and between laboratories, as opposed to random error (imprecision). Quoting Büttner again: "For clinical chemistry, in 1974 Westgard and coworkers proposed a total error concept. Because of its simplicity, such a concept has indisputable advantages in daily practice, for instance in defining and monitoring the achievement of performance goals for laboratories. On the other hand, it makes it more difficult to clearly detect a bias in routine laboratories. Specification of a total error tends to conceal the lack of trueness as a methodological problem."[12] Clearly, trueness must be assessed to comprehend the total error inherent in an analytical procedure.

METROLOGICAL TRACEABILITY

The in vitro diagnostics (IVD) Directive (IVDD; 98/79/EC), approved by European Union Parliament in October 1998, and effective December 7, 2003, states in Essential Requirements/General Requirements/Item 3, paragraph 2: "The traceability of values assigned to calibrators and ... (trueness) control materials must be assured through available reference measurement procedures and/or available reference materials of a higher order."[13] The IVDD states "controls" and makes no distinction between precision and accuracy controls. De Leer and Lequin[13] make it clear that the IVDD addresses accuracy controls, and is not applicable to control materials that do not have an assigned value and are used only for assessing the precision of a measurement procedure, either its repeatability or reproducibility, in other words, precision controls. Although the IVDD calls for traceability, it does not describe how to establish traceability but instead points to International Organization for Standardization (ISO) 17511, In vitro diagnostic medical devices—Measurement of quantities in samples of biologic origin—Metrological traceability of values assigned to calibrators and control materials.[14] **Fig. 1** illustrates a generic metrological traceability flowchart for

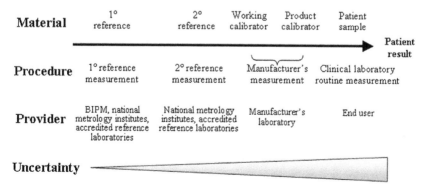

Fig. 1. A generic calibrator traceability flowchart. (*From* Armbruster D, Miller RR. The Joint Committee for Traceability in Laboratory Medicine (JCTLM): a global approach to promote the standardisation of clinical laboratory test results. Clin Biochem Rev 2007;28:105–14; with permission.)

an assay calibrator. The patient test results are traceable back to reference materials and/or methods of the highest metrological order available. ISO 17511 states "It is essential that results reported to physicians and patients are adequately accurate (true and precise) to allow correct medical interpretation and comparability over time and space." Clearly, 17511 calls for accuracy controls as both trueness/bias and precision must be assessed. ISO 17511 notes that some analytes (often called Type A) have both reference materials and methods (eg, electrolytes and glucose), or only a reference method (eg, enzymes), or neither a reference material or method (eg, tumor markers). These latter analytes are often called Type B.

Accuracy controls must conform to ISO 17511, and for enzymes, ISO 18153 (In vitro diagnostic medical devices—Measurement of quantities in biologic samples—Metrological traceability of values for catalytic concentration of enzymes assigned to calibrators and control materials). Without metrological traceability to a reference measurement system (RMS), patient test results for the same patient from different laboratories may not be comparable, a major expectation of the electronic medical record (EMR). This poses an increasingly relevant problem to the practice of modern clinical laboratory medicine as the use of the EMR becomes more common.

Powers[15] states that "The traceability of values assigned to calibrators and/or control materials must be assumed to be traceable through available reference measurement procedures and/or available reference materials of higher order" but also notes that "demonstrating traceability is not the same as demonstrating accuracy." Powers[15] explains a significant distinction between the European and US perspective: "The new regulatory requirements for calibrator traceability have largely been driven by the comparatively greater importance northern European laboratory professionals place on accuracy, which they believe is essential to the transferability of patients' results from laboratory to laboratory and country to country…Whereas US laboratories accept differences among methods as inevitable and compensate with method-specific reference ranges, their European counterparts have refused to abandon the pursuit of analytical truth."

The distinction between the traditional precision controls and the growing interest in and the need for accuracy controls spills over into external quality assessment/proficiency testing (EQA/PT) programs. As Büttner writes: "… in the proficiency testing, so called 'peer group mean values' are employed as target values, and these do not lead to any improvement of the trueness or therefore of the comparability."[12] To promote comparability of test results, EQA/PT samples must be traceable as per 17511 and have target values against which laboratories are graded on the basis of absolute accuracy ("scientific truth" as determined by a reference material or method), as opposed to peer group grading, which provides only a relative measure of accuracy.

COMMUTABILITY

"A fundamental goal of laboratory medicine is that results for patients' samples will be comparable independent of the medical laboratory that produced the results."[16] Among other considerations, this requires commutability of reference materials, such as accuracy controls. As explained previously, commutability is defined as the consistency of the relationship between results obtained by different analytical methods for reference materials, such as an accuracy control and patient specimens. Commutability is the property that determines if the concentration of an analyte measured by a field method is equivalent to that obtained by reference method analysis. A sample may be commutable with many field methods but not with all, therefore commutability is a relative instead of an absolute property and must be confirmed with any given method. Commutability of an accuracy control can be determined only experimentally with a designated field method. If a control is commutable, the control results from a reference method and field methods should be directly comparable. Lack of commutability for a control when tested using a reference method and a field method is attributable to a lack of trueness (ie, there is a bias between the methods).

Controls, whether precision or accuracy, are intended to monitor the analytical process as surrogates for patient specimens. It is appropriate that controls are prepared in a matrix that mimics human serum, plasma, or other body fluids. The lack of commutability for reference materials and controls is usually referred to as a matrix effect, and has been shown to be a common problem.[16] The matrix effect is defined as "the influence of a property of the sample, other than the measurand, on the measurement of the measurand according to a specified measurement procedure and thereby on its measured value."[14] The term "matrix effect" is sometimes erroneously used for the lack of commutability due to a denatured analyte or an added nongenuine component ("surrogate analyte") meant to simulate the analyte. The Clinical Laboratory Standards Institute (CLSI)/ISO-harmonized terminology defines matrix as the totality of components of a material system except the analyte.

As noted by Ross and colleagues,[3] commenting on a study to assess trueness in proficiency testing, "Because of matrix biases, the reference value was the correct target value only 32% of the time; thus, the traceability established by definitive method and reference method value assignments on Chemistry Survey specimens did not assure accuracy on patient samples." For 1971 and 1972 College of American Pathologists (CAP) surveys, it was noted that "... the chemical interactions of lyophilized specimens may not be exactly comparable to the reactions of fresh human serum," and that "accuracy measurements always carry the risk that a bias stems from some feature of the specimens used for the study and that this bias would not be apparent in fresh patient material."

The need for commutability was a cause for the publication of CLSI Guideline C37, Preparation and validation of commutable frozen human serum pools as secondary reference materials for cholesterol measurement procedures.[17] A Dutch study demonstrated the superior quality of native samples in comparison with the regular samples used by EQA programs and underscores the need for fresh native sera as the first choice for use as EQA samples.[18] As a result of this study, the Dutch EQA program replaced the regular samples with commutable fresh frozen sera in all regular chemistry EQA surveys after 2004. In addition, when feasible, value assignment is made using reference methods, allowing for accuracy-based grading instead of inferior peer-group grading. Quam[19] also recommends that native samples that are commutable should be used as trueness controls in EQA schemes.

Calibration traceability does not ensure trueness of measured values for patient samples, owing to potential lack of commutability, that is, equivalent results may not be obtained with patient samples when different routine (field) methods are compared, even if all methods use calibrators traceable to the same higher order references, especially for Type B measurands.[20]

PRECISION VERSUS ACCURACY CONTROLS

Testing QC samples is standard practice in the clinical laboratory as part of a quality assurance system, but testing controls is not the same thing as controlling quality. Quality assurance is an all-inclusive system for monitoring the accuracy of test results, incorporating all steps: preanalytical, analytical, and postanalytical. QC is the system used to monitor analytical performance. QC is used to detect analytical errors and prevent reporting of erroneous test results. Traditionally, QC monitors only precision by assaying precision controls. Control metrics consist of the mean value, the SD, and %CV. QC results typically are reported as %CV. The %CV is an estimate of precision, but an acceptable %CV does not necessarily mean that results are accurate because it does not reflect trueness/bias. If a precision control exceeds the acceptance limit, it is not known to what extent the failure is attributable to random and systematic error, as only random error is considered.

Precision controls are assayed or nonassayed. Nonassayed controls have no set target value and laboratories determine the mean values themselves. Assayed controls have assigned target values; however, the target values of assayed controls are usually the means of various analyzers/methods, not trueness target values assigned by reference method analysis, which would be applicable for any analyzer and method. Although it is generally assumed that QC reflects accuracy, accuracy, by definition, includes both precision and trueness (bias) and precision controls assess only precision.

As noted by Mitchell,[1] present QC schemes tend to monitor only precision, or at best accuracy based on the findings of other laboratories. All participant mean values produce only a "state-of-the art value," but a "definitive" approach measures the concentration of a measurand that gives results that are accepted as the nearest attainable to the true value, that is, accuracy based on an established reference method (eg, Ca measured by isotope dilution-mass spectrometry [ID-MS]).

As opposed to precision controls, accuracy control values should be traceable to "truth," as determined by reference materials and/or methods. Accuracy controls are special control materials intended to assess "trueness of measurement." Accuracy controls may also be called trueness controls, but analysis of these controls will inherently involve an RE component (imprecision) in addition to the SE component (trueness, bias). "Accuracy control" seems more appropriate given the accepted definition of accuracy, which includes both precision and trueness. Routine controls used to verify the consistency over time of routine measurement procedures and reliability of laboratory testing systems usually do not conform to ISO 17511 or ISO 18153. Metrological traceability is possible for many routine analytes, such as the electrolytes, creatinine, urea, uric acid, glucose, and cholesterol, but is considerably more difficult for more complex analytes, usually those measured by immunometric procedures, such as thyroid and tumor markers and fertility hormones. Production of accuracy controls is more complicated and costly than precision controls because target values must be assigned by recognized reference method analysis or by weighing in reference material into a commutable matrix. Creating accuracy controls for more complex analytes is even more difficult because these analytes are not well characterized and neither reference materials nor methods may be available. Enzymes represent a special case, as it is the concentration of enzyme catalytic activity that is measured instead of analyte concentration expressed in mass units. Reference methods have been developed by the IFCC for the more common enzymes and accuracy controls can be provided for enzymes by analyzing them using the internationally accepted reference methods, but production of large quantities of enzyme accuracy controls poses logistical difficulties.

Typical QC is used to assess precision, but not accuracy, because of the lack of a traceable target value assigned to controls. To truly assess accuracy, it may be necessary to use one control for precision and another for trueness/bias, unless a true accuracy control is used, one that monitors both bias and precision.

An accuracy control could be a secondary reference material or a standard, or a control that is manufactured in the same fashion as a reference material or standard. A primary reference standard is prepared from a precisely weighed analyte that is put into solution, but the matrix may be aqueous. Even if serum or plasma is used as the matrix, the material may not be commutable. A secondary standard has a target value assigned against the primary standard and/or reference procedure and is prepared in a commutable matrix to mimic a patient sample. An accuracy control, as a secondary reference material, may be less accurate than a primary reference standard or calibrator, in the sense that the uncertainty of the target value may be greater, but should also be less expensive and more readily available and so more suitable for use in the clinical laboratory. A key requirement is that an accuracy control demonstrates commutability, that is, its analytical response is the same as a fresh patient specimen when tested by a reference method and a field method.

PRACTICAL GUIDANCE FOR USE OF ACCURACY CONTROLS

The challenge for the typical clinical laboratory is to find a suitable accuracy control and how to incorporate it into its QC scheme. Most control providers do not offer accuracy controls and laboratories must look to institutes of metrology or other organizations that provide reference materials. CLSI EP15 (Evaluation Protocol), User Verification of Performance for Precision and Trueness, suggests sources of reference materials that can be used as accuracy controls.[21] They include certified reference materials from the National Institutes of Standards and Technology and the Joint Committee for Traceability in Laboratory Medicine (JCTLM) database of reference materials (JCTLM.org), EQA/PT programs, assay manufacturers, and third-party providers. The JCTLM has approved a large number of reference materials that could be used as accuracy controls and lists the contract information for the providers. Some EQA/PT programs also offer commutable samples with target values assigned by reference methods (samples used in EQA/PT programs that use accuracy-based grading, as opposed to peer group grading). The CAP, for example, provides samples for Hb A1c and creatinine that are suitable for use as accuracy controls. Other potential sources include the UK National External Quality Assessment Service and the Royal College of Pathologists of Australasia. Companies that sell products intended to be used for calibration verification and linearity may also be sources for accuracy controls. Unfortunately, acceptable accuracy controls are simply not available for the wide spectrum of analytes measured in the clinical laboratory.

EP15 explains that trueness/bias may be verified by comparability (split sample comparison; results from 2 methods compared, to determine if a significant difference exists), or recovery of expected values from certified reference materials.[21] The comparability approach is not optimal because it involves 2 field methods and there is no guarantee that the one designated as the "reference method" is truly accurate. Recovery of assigned target values for reference materials is necessary. Of course, for valid verification of accuracy, the reference material must be commutable. Preferably, 2 accuracy controls will be tested, spanning the dynamic range of an assay, or controls with target concentrations at clinically significant concentrations (medical decision levels) will be used. Measuring the controls in duplicate and over 2 or more analytical runs is recommended. The laboratory must decide the acceptance limit for an accuracy control, perhaps using a statistical limit or a clinical interpretation specification. Under the TEa concept, bias limits are available for many analytes.

Even though suitable accuracy controls are often not readily available, laboratories should implement their use when feasible to assess the trueness/bias of their assays. Ideally, daily use of an accuracy control that monitors both RE (precision) and SE (bias) would be used. As noted previously, the limited ready availability of accuracy control materials, and the cost of such materials, likely makes this unfeasible for the typical clinical laboratory. Testing of available accuracy controls on a routine basis, perhaps weekly or monthly, is practical. Although less than optimal, periodic use of accuracy controls would be an improvement on the usual state of affairs in the clinical laboratory, as regular assessment of trueness/bias rarely occurs except on initial validation/verification testing for a new method or when a laboratory is enrolled in one of the few available accuracy-based EQA/PT surveys.

Büttner's[12] observations from 1995 still hold true: "The recognition that today it is not so much the precision as the trueness of the analysis which requires improvement in laboratory medicine …," "… reference materials have exact values for specific properties. These values may therefore be employed as 'conventional true values' for examining the accuracy and in particular the trueness of routine analysis methods," and "finally, a correct assessment of the performance of medical laboratories is not possible within quality control schemes if accuracy is not made the primary goal." If accuracy is truly the goal, then accuracy controls, which measure both bias and precision, must be used.

ROLE OF PROVIDERS OF REFERENCE MATERIALS AND IVD REAGENT MANUFACTURERS

Reference materials and control samples should be characterized by their providers and manufacturers and clearly described as either suitable for use as precision controls or accuracy controls. The metrological traceability of accuracy controls should be fully described by providing an unbroken chain of value transfers, as depicted by the flowchart in **Fig. 1**. Accuracy control values should generally be set at MDLs or other appropriate clinically significant concentrations. Providers should distinguish between a standard or calibrator and a control because standards/calibrators should not be used as controls, nor should controls be used as standards/calibrators. Third party controls are preferred to controls from the same manufacturer that produces the calibrators for an assay, as they provide an independent, unbiased assessment of performance. When using the same manufacturer as the source for controls and calibrators, it may be that the materials have been produced in the same way and may show consistent performance, even when the testing process has changed. In fact, the Food and Drug Administration issued a note of caution about using only control materials supplied by the instrument manufacturer after problems with analytic systems in US laboratories.[19] Laboratories were advised to include control materials made by companies other than the instrument manufacturer to provide better assurance that methods are performing properly.

A practical example of why accuracy controls are desirable is demonstrated by the results of a study to assess the accuracy of glucose measured by clinical laboratories in Korea.[22] Korean laboratories using the common field methods for glucose (oxidase-peroxidase, glucose oxidase by electrode, glucose oxidase dry chemistry method, and glucose-6-phosphate dehydrogenase [G6PD] methods) tested reference materials (RMs) for glucose, which are not in widespread use because of the high cost and limited availability. These secondary RMs were prepared from commutable frozen human serum pools to evaluate the accuracy of the glucose field methods. Pools were prepared from surplus serum spiked with glucose powder and stored at -70°C. Pools of 5 concentrations with uncertainties were assayed by 2 reference methods listed by the JCTLM (ID-MS and G6PD) and target values for each pool were assigned. The RMs were shown to be commutable with the field methods by acceptable agreement with reference method target values.[23] Diabetes diagnosis uses 2 cutoffs, 7.0 mmol/L (126 mg/dL) and 11.1 mmol/L (200 mg/dL), and accurate glucose results are of course essential for correct classification of patients. Guidelines call for precision to be less than 3.3%, bias to be less than 2.5%, and TE to be less than 7.9%. Twelve proficiency testing (PT) samples were prepared from lyophilized human serum RMs and value assigned by isotope dilution-gas chromatography/mass spectrometry (ID-GC/MS), the accepted reference method. Samples were sent to about 700 laboratories, 95% of which used the hexokinase or glucose oxidase methods for glucose. Only 47% of results had bias less than 2.5%, the maximum allowable bias, in comparison with the reference method target values (36.6% for glucose oxidase; 49.6% for hexokinase). Although lyophilization might have caused a matrix effect, the mean %CV was less than 5% and there was a positive mean bias of 2% compared with the RMP target value.[23] These findings required the use of PT samples that were suitable for use as accuracy controls. Some field methods were capable of meeting the bias goal for glucose, but others were not. If accuracy controls were readily available, laboratories could routinely monitor their own performance. Because such controls are uncommon, manufacturers are obligated to assess the performance of their products in terms of both precision and trueness/bias.

Trueness must be primarily addressed by manufacturers, as it is not feasible for clinical laboratories to routinely assess bias without making special efforts. And traceability needs to be ensured by manufacturers, as few clinical laboratories have the time and resources to do it. Confirming commutability of accuracy controls is also a responsibility of manufacturers. To quote Miller,[16] "Providers of reference and trueness control materials that are intended for calibration or routine measurement procedures (or for assessment of calibration status) must include commutability validation as an essential requirement. Good laboratory practice requires that reference materials intended for measurement with routine procedures be provided with commutability information included in the certificate of analysis or product labeling."

For manufacturers, the definitions of verification and validation discussed previously are key. Verification by a manufacturer confirms that an assay meets specified analytical performance requirements (ie, the manufacturer has "built the test right"). But validation testing is necessary to prove that assay's performance, including accuracy, is adequate for its intended use (ie, the manufacturer has "built the right test"). Accuracy controls should be manufactured in the same manner as calibrators and be used for verification and validation testing.

As stated by Westgard,[8] trueness must be addressed to achieve quality and it requires traceability of reference materials and accuracy controls. Trueness, and thus, ultimately, accuracy, must be primarily addressed by manufacturers. Thienpont[24] also calls on manufacturers to take the lead: "Ideally, the driving force should be the test providers, being industry or laboratories developing assays. Frankly, the author hoped some years ago that one of the major players would announce a new measurement paradigm in clinical chemistry, namely, to move toward accuracy-based assays and demonstrate transparency by comparing assays with accepted reference measurement procedures." Few health care laboratories have the time and resources to establish traceability and ensure accuracy. In the clinical laboratory, the only practical approach is for those assays for which certified reference materials are available to be properly traceable using the concepts of metrology to ensure appropriate calibration of methods and trueness of patient test results. The practical measure is bias, which is inherent in the systematic concept of accuracy, through the concept of TEa.

REFERENCES

1. Mitchell FL. Quality control in clinical chemistry. Proc R Soc Med 1975;68:613–5.
2. Caraway WT. Accuracy in clinical chemistry. Clin Chem 1971;17:63–71.

3. Ross JW, Miller WG, Myers GL, et al. The accuracy of laboratory measurements in clinical chemistry. Arch Pathol Lab Med 1998;122:587–608.
4. Armbruster D, Miller RR. The Joint Committee for Traceability in Laboratory Medicine (JCTLM): a global approach to promote the standardisation of clinical laboratory test results. Clin Biochem Rev 2007;28:105–14.
5. Bruns D, Oosterhuis WP. Evidence-based guidelines in laboratory medicine: principles and methods. In: Price CP, Christenson RH, editors. Evidence-based laboratory medicine: from principles to outcomes. Washington, DC: AACC Press; 2003. p. 201.
6. Rosenbaum JM. Accuracy in clinical laboratories participating in regional quality control programs. Arch Pathol Lab Med 1985;109:485–95.
7. International Bureau of Weights and Measures (BIPM). International vocabulary of metrology—basic and general concepts and associated terms (VIM). 3rd edition. Joint Committee for Guides in Metrology (JCGM). France: Pavillon de Breteuil; 2012.
8. Westgard JO. Basic method validation. 3rd edition. Madison (WI): Westgard QC; 2008. p. 23, 257.
9. Eisenhart C. Expression of the uncertainties if final results. Science 1968;160: 1201.
10. Westgard JO, Darcy T. The truth about quality: medical usefulness and analytical reliability of laboratory tests. Clin Chim Acta 2004;346:3–11.
11. Westgard JO, Barry PL. Cost-effective quality control: managing the quality and productivity of analytical processes. Washington, DC: AACC Press; 2006. p. 41–2.
12. Büttner J. The need for accuracy in clinical chemistry. Eur J Clin Chem Clin Biochem 1995;33:981–8.
13. De Leer WB, Lequin RM. The European in-vitro diagnostic medical devices directive: it's implications of the clinical marketplace and healthcare measurements standards. J Lab Autom 2000;5:66–8.
14. International Organization for Standardization (ISO) 17511, in vitro diagnostic medical devices—Measurement of quantities in samples of biological origin—Metrological traceability of values assigned to calibrators and control materials. ISO/prEN 17511. Geneva (IL): International Organization for Standardization; 1999.
15. Powers DM. Traceability of assay calibrators: the EU's IVD directive raises the bar. IVD Technology 2000;24:26–33.
16. Miller WG, Myers GL, Rej R. Why commutability matters. Clin Chem 2006;52: 553–4.
17. Clinical and Laboratory Standards Institute (CLSI) C37A, Preparation and validation of commutable frozen human serum pools as secondary reference materials for cholesterol measurement procedures. Wayne (PA): Clinical Laboratory Standards Institute; 1999.
18. Baadenhuijsen H, Kuypers A, Weykamp C, et al. External quality assessment in the Netherlands: time to introduce commutable survey specimens. Lessons from the Dutch "Calibration 2000" project. Clin Chem Lab Med 2005;43:304–7.
19. Quam EF. QC - The materials. In: Westgard JO, editor. Basic QC practices. 3rd edition. Madison (WI): Westgard QC; 2010. p. 168.
20. Sturgeon CM, Berger P, Bidart JM, et al. Differences in recognition of the 1st WHO International Reference Reagents for hCG-related isoforms by diagnostic immunoassays for human chorionic gonadotropin. Clin Chem 2009;55: 1484–91.

21. Clinical and Laboratory Standards Institute (CLSI) EP15A2, User verification of performance for precision and trueness. Wayne (PA): Clinical Laboratory Standards Institute; 2005.

22. Lee W, Chung HJ, Hannestad U, et al. Trueness assessment of Korean nationwide glucose proficiency testing. Clin Chem Lab Med 2011;49:1061–4.

23. Xia C, Liu O, Wang L, et al. Trueness assessment for serum glucose measurement using commercial systems through preparation of commutable reference materials. Ann Lab Med 2012;32:243–9.

24. Thienpont LM. Accuracy in clinical chemistry—who will kiss sleeping beauty awake? Clin Chem Lab Med 2008;46:1220–2.

Patient Population Controls

R. Neill Carey, PhD, FACB

KEYWORDS

- Quality control • Average of normals • Patient data • Patient population controls

KEY POINTS

- QC procedures incorporating AoN algorithms can extend run length with objective decisions about the acceptability of performance between reference sample control observations.
- Incorporating AoN algorithms into QC procedures can significantly improve the overall error detection for some low sigma methods.
- Applicability of an AoN algorithm to the QC procedure for a particular test depends on the s_{pop}/s_{meas} ratio for the test, the volume of patient samples available to an individual instrument performing the test, the width of the control limits, and the distribution of outlying patient results.
- "One size fits all" does not apply to QC procedures incorporating AoN algorithms. Each test's AoN procedure must be tailored to its characteristics. Access to power function graphs or QC planning software is required.
- QC procedures incorporating AoN algorithms are not sensitive to random error.

EVOLUTION OF PATIENT POPULATION CONTROLS

With the development of quality control (QC) plans based on risk management, it is expected that laboratories will combine different types of controls to monitor different failure modes or different sources of errors. Addition of patient controls is attractive to laboratories because they make use of the results from routine testing of patient samples and are, in a sense, free controls. The real question is whether they are cost-effective, which must also consider their effectiveness for detecting medically important errors.

In traditional reference sample QC, samples are typically tested at scheduled times, depending on the definition of an analytical run. Testing may be done once daily for a very stable method, or as often as every few hours for an unstable method. If the controls tested at the start of the defined time period and those tested at the end of the period are within acceptable limits, the patient testing has been bracketed, and one assumes that performance was stable for the entire period. It is taken on faith that the testing process has been stable because both sets of controls were acceptable. For objective evidence that the process was stable, it must be monitored

104 Elizabeth Street, Salisbury, MD 21801, USA
E-mail address: rogernc1@msn.com

Clin Lab Med 33 (2013) 139–146
http://dx.doi.org/10.1016/j.cll.2012.11.002
0272-2712/13/$ – see front matter © 2013 Elsevier Inc. All rights reserved.

between the controls. QC procedures based on patient results can provide a monitoring function in many situations.

If a patient population is stable, the mean value of the population of results for a particular analyte are stable. There may be large variation in the mean when only a few patient results are averaged, but the mean stabilizes as more patient results are averaged. When the mean of many patient results varies significantly from its established value, a change in the process (shift or drift) may have occurred.

QC procedures using the means of patient populations, or "average of normals" (AoN) algorithms, are well established, beginning with their description by Hoffman and Waid in 1965.[1] AoN procedures first became widely used in hematology laboratories, where they were implemented on multichannel automated hematology cell counters to monitor the averages of patients' red cell indices. Hematology laboratories typically use multistage QC procedures consisting of a startup with traditional QC materials, and then monitoring with a combination of AoN (Bull's algorithm[2]) and retained patient specimens.[3] These procedures provide error detection capability during the periods between testing of QC materials, improve overall error detection capability, and result in lowered usage of expensive QC materials.

Initially, the application of AoN monitoring procedures for chemistry tests was limited to large laboratories with customized computer software capabilities. More recently, laboratory middleware products have implemented software to provide AoN algorithms, and usage of AoN procedures has become more widespread.

Calculation of control limits for AoN procedures is more complicated than it is for reference sample QC. When the mean is calculated for a batch of patient samples, control limits can be calculated as confidence limits around the grand mean. More typically, patient means and control limits are calculated by exponential smoothing techniques.[4]

PERFORMANCE CHARACTERISTICS OF AON QC PROCEDURES

Cembrowski and colleagues[4,5] and Westgard and colleagues[6] have extensively studied the performance of AoN procedures through computer simulation. Together these reports describe the behavior of AoN procedures for a wide variety of tests, and provide numerous example power function curves. The significant factors for predicting performance of AoN procedures found in the two studies are summarized next, in decreasing order of importance.

- Ratio of the patient population standard deviation to the method's analytical standard deviation, s_{pop}/s_{meas}: As the patient population standard deviation decreases relative to the method's analytical standard deviation, each patient result becomes more like a control result. For tests such as sodium and chloride, for which s_{pop} values are only a few multiples of s_{meas} (typical s_{pop}/s_{meas} ratios are 1.5–3.0), only 10 to 20 patient results need to be averaged for the AoN procedure to perform similarly to multirule QC procedures with two controls. For some of these low ratio tests, AoN QC procedures can complement, and even may outperform, traditional reference sample QC. For tests with large s_{pop}/s_{meas} ratios, even averaging several hundred patient test results may not yield satisfactory error detection. Cembrowski and colleagues[5] summarized this behavior in a nomogram illustrating the sensitivity of AoN procedures to detect a shift of 2 s_{meas} as a function of the number of samples averaged for s_{pop}/s_{meas} ratios of 2 to 10 when P_{fr} is 0.01 or 1%.
- The number of samples averaged, N_p: As more samples are averaged, the population variation is averaged out, limits tighten, and the AoN procedure becomes

more sensitive to shifts. Cembrowski and colleagues[5] demonstrated this effect in the form of a nomogram illustrating the relationship between the number of samples averaged (N_p), s_{pop}/s_{meas}, and P_{ed} for a shift of two s_{meas}. Westgard and colleagues[6] presented OPSpecs charts and power function curves for two example tests with s_{pop}/s_{meas} ratios of 5 and 9, respectively, with N_p ranging from 20 to 450.

- Width of the control limits: As P_{fr} decreases (wider limits), sensitivity to shifts decreases. If the reference sample QC procedure is weak, more sensitivity is needed from the AoN procedure, and P_{fr} could be set higher, if it can be tolerated.
- Truncation limits and the population beyond truncation limits: Outliers reduce the sensitivity of AoN for tests with high s_{pop}/s_{meas} ratios more than for tests with low s_{pop}/s_{meas} ratios. A truncation limit of 3 s_{pop} seems reasonable for most populations. It may be best to exclude patient populations that are expected to have a high percentage of outliers, such as emergency department patients.

Both studies included summary tables of population mean, s_{pop}, s_{meas}, and s_{pop}/s_{meas} values for tests having s_{pop}/s_{meas} ratios from 1.7 to 23.

Westgard and Stein[7] added AoN capability software to a QC planning program that can automatically (or manually) select QC procedures to maintain a stated level of quality, based on input parameters, such as allowable error, s_{meas}, bias, expected instability, number of control replicates, and s_{pop}/s_{meas}. AoN procedures were described as tools for maximizing run length because they can objectively signal the presence or absence of systematic error in the interval between scheduled testing of control materials. The QC planning program was used to propose optimal AoN procedures for the 38 example tests from a regional reference laboratory in a summary table that included population statistics, daily patient testing volumes, test characteristics, and quality planning parameters (including P_{ed}) for design of AoN algorithms. The authors concluded that control of approximately half of the tests studied could be improved significantly by use of AoN procedures to monitor run length.

Westgard[8] used the same set of examples with the current version of the QC planning software (EZ Rules 3; Westgard QC, Madison, WI) to further illustrate the capabilities of AoN procedures in general and to demonstrate how they can provide better control for some low sigma, low s_{pop}/s_{meas} methods than reference sample QC. For several methods with sigma values between 2.5 and 4.5, AoN procedures would provide P_{ed} higher than 0.90 or a 90% chance of detecting critically sized errors with P_{fr} of nearly zero, with between 30 and 120 patient results averaged. For sodium, chloride, and calcium, which are difficult to control with reference sample QC, P_{ed} values higher than 0.90 were achieved for ΔSE_{Crit} with 30, 60, and 60 patient results, respectively. These successes are explained by the respective s_{pop}/s_{meas} ratios of 1.6, 2.6, and 1.8. However, some low sigma tests with high s_{pop}/s_{meas} ratios could not be controlled by AoN even with groups of 300 to 600 patient samples.

The results and conclusions of the Cembrowski and Westgard investigations were based on computer simulations to estimate P_{ed} and P_{fr} with the goal of maximizing P_{ed} and minimizing P_{fr}.[4,5] Ye and colleagues[9] performed simulations of AoN performance to estimate the average number of patient results reported between the inception of an error condition and its detection (ANP_{ed}), and the average number of patient results in that group with errors exceeding allowable error (ANP_{TE}). Six analytes were studied (calcium, potassium, sodium, cholesterol, total protein, and aspartate aminotransferase [AST]). When systematic errors were small, increasing the number of patient results decreased ANP_{ed} (increasing sensitivity, as found in previous studies). However, when systematic errors were large, decreasing the numbers of patient results averaged decreased ANP_{ed} and ANP_{TE} (because detection was quicker). The worst-case ANP_{TE} occurred at a median systematic error 1.4 s_{meas} greater than allowable error, which would be about 3 s_{meas} higher than the ΔSE_{Crit} that is critical to detect in the Westgard model.

The difference in critical error levels to control between the Cembrowski-Westgard and Ye models seems significant; however, it may not make much of a practical difference because most of the AoN monitoring is done continuously by exponential smoothing or other forms of running means. Although the calculated means represent the stated number of patient results, the calculations give more weight to the most recent results. This satisfies the need to average many data for high P_{ed}, and to be more responsive to systematic error in recent data.

SELECTION OF AON QC PROCEDURES FOR A SPECIFIC TEST

Selecting the optimal AoN procedure is not trivial. Westgard[8] and Cembrowski and Carey[4] give advice on how to go about it.

- Study the population of patient results, and determine its mean and s_{pop}. Use patient results accumulated during a period of several months, if possible. Remove outliers beyond 3 s_{pop} limits and recalculate s_{pop}. It is critical to use patient results from one's own institution's population. s_{pop}/s_{meas} ratios can vary widely among different populations; for example, Cembrowski reported an s_{pop}/s_{meas} of 2.9 for total bilirubin, whereas Westgard and colleagues reported an s_{pop}/s_{meas} of 8.6.
- Determine s_{meas} for a control material whose mean concentration is close to the trimmed patient mean. Calculate s_{pop}/s_{meas}.
- Calculate ΔSE_{Crit} for the control material from allowable error, s_{meas}, and bias, if any.
- Examine power function curves for candidate AoN procedures and select the optimal procedure as the one that provides P_{ed} greater than 0.90 or 90% probability of detecting critically sized errors with the lowest number of patients averaged and acceptable P_{fr}. It may be impossible to achieve this P_{ed} for tests with high s_{pop}/s_{meas}, or for tests with low daily volumes of patient testing; however, even an AoN procedure with P_{ed} of 0.50 for ΔSE_{Crit} provides monitoring between controls and lessens the risk that large errors go undetected.

EXAMPLE APPLICATIONS OF AON CONTROL PROCEDURES

The process of selecting an AoN procedure is demonstrated next with examples for chloride, albumin, creatinine, and urea nitrogen. These analytes are of particular interest for monitoring dialysis patients, and AoN procedures should be applicable in specialized laboratories that support renal dialysis centers.

Chloride

$\overline{X}_{pop}$ = 103.6 mmol/L; s_{pop} = 3.46 mmol/L; s_{meas} = 1.21 mmol/L (CV = 1.17%); s_{pop}/s_{meas} = 2.9; and CLIA allowable total error = 5%. Sigma is 4.27 and ΔSE_{Crit} is 2.62. At startup, four control replicates have P_{ed} for ΔSE_{Crit} of 0.94 or 94% detection with the $1_{2.5s}$ rule. For run length control, an AoN procedure with N_p = 30 provides P_{ed} of 0.91 for ΔSE_{Crit} with P_{fr} near zero, as documented by the power function graph (or sigma-metric QC selection graph) in **Fig. 1**. The different curves from top to bottom correspond to averages of 100, 60, 40, 30, 20, and 10 patient samples (N_p). The fourth curve from the top corresponds to 30 patient samples and its intersection with the vertical

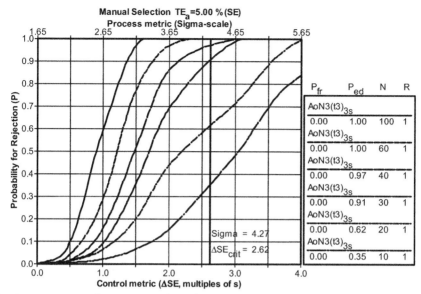

Fig. 1. Power curves for AoN procedures for chloride where CLIA TEa is 5%, method CV is 1.17%, and s_{pop}/s_{meas} ratio is 3. Minimum number of patient samples should be 30, as shown by fourth curve from the top.

line (for sigma = 4.27 and ΔSE_{Crit} is 2.62) shows the expected P_{ed} (0.91). The y-intercept of this curve shows the expected P_{fr} (0.00). This volume of testing should easily be reached on a single instrument in less than an hour in a medium-sized hospital laboratory during the day, and probably over a shift on evenings, nights, and weekends.

Albumin

$\overline{X}_{pop}$ = 3.9 g/dL; s_{pop} = 0.44 g/dL; s_{meas} = 0.08 g/dL (CV = 2.05%); s_{pop}/s_{meas} = 5.5; and CLIA allowable total error = 10%. Sigma is 4.88 and ΔSE_{Crit} is 3.23. At startup, two control replicates have P_{ed} for ΔSE_{Crit} of 0.92 with the $1_{2.5s}$ rule. For run length control, an AoN procedure with N_p = 90 provides P_{ed} of 0.99, as shown by the second curve from the top in the power function graph in **Fig. 2**. A laboratory whose patient albumin testing volume on a single instrument does not reach 90 in a reasonable time could consider N_p = 60 where P_{ed} for ΔSE_{Crit} is 0.84, as shown by the third curve from the top.

Creatinine

$\overline{X}_{pop}$ = 0.89 mg/dL; s_{pop} = 0.28 mg/dL; s_{meas} = 0.07 mg/dL (CV = 7.9%); s_{pop}/s_{meas} = 4; and CLIA allowable error = 0.3 mg/dL (33.7%). Sigma is 4.27 and ΔSE_{Crit} is 2.62. At startup, four control replicates have P_{ed} for ΔSE_{Crit} of 0.94 with the $1_{2.5s}$ rule. For run length control, an AoN procedure with N_p = 60 provides P_{ed} of 0.94, as shown by the third curve from the top in **Fig. 3**.

Urea Nitrogen

$\overline{X}_{pop}$ = 14.5 mg/dL; s_{pop} = 5.46 mg/dL; s_{meas} = 0.42 mg/dL (CV = 2.9%); s_{pop}/s_{meas} = 13; and allowable error = 2.0 mg/dL. Sigma is 4.76 and ΔSE_{Crit} is 3.11. At startup, four control replicates have P_{ed} for ΔSE_{Crit} of 0.93 with the $1_{2.5s}$ rule. For the AoN procedure,

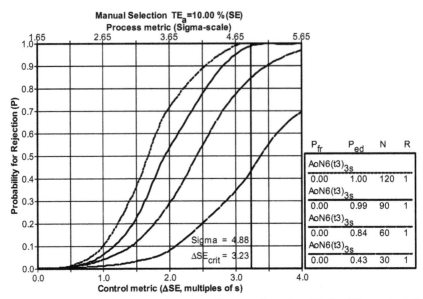

Fig. 2. Power curves for AoN procedures for albumin where CLIA TEa is 10%, method CV is 2.05%, and s_{pop}/s_{meas} ratio is 6. Minimum number of patient samples should be 90, as shown by second curve from the top.

as shown in **Fig. 4**, 300 patient samples must be averaged from a single instrument to achieve P_{ed} of 0.84 or 84% detection for ΔSE_{Crit}, or 180 patient samples to have P_{ed} of 0.53 or 53% detection. Only large laboratories have such large volumes of patient testing on a single instrument in a reasonable time.

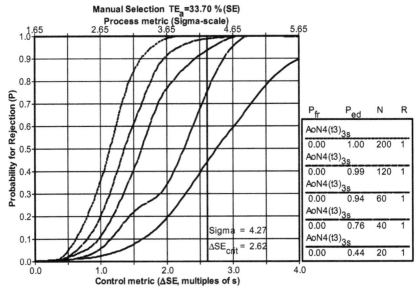

Fig. 3. Power curves for AoN procedures for creatinine where CLIA TEa is 0.3 mg/dL (or 33.7% at 0.89 mg/dL); method CV is 7.9%; and s_{pop}/s_{meas} ratio is 4. Minimum number of patient samples should be 60, as shown by third curve from the top.

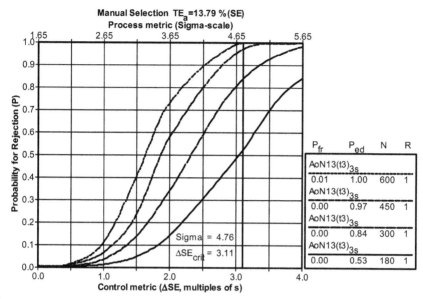

Fig. 4. Power curves for AoN procedures for urea nitrogen where CLIA TEa is 2 mg/dL (or 13.79% at 14.5 mg/dL); method CV is 2.9%; and s_{pop}/s_{meas} ratio is 13. Minimum number of patient samples should be between 450 and 300, as shown by second and third curves from the top.

These examples demonstrate how some tests can benefit from use of AoN procedures. Of the 38 tests examined by Westgard and colleagues[6] in a regional laboratory, 13 would benefit from AoN procedures with N_p of 100 or less, with P_{ed} for ΔSE_{Crit} of 0.90 or more. Eleven would require larger N_p and 14 had low P_{ed} for ΔSE_{Crit} with the number of samples available.

A FEW GENERAL CAVEATS ABOUT AON PROCEDURES

AoN procedures are not sensitive to random error, and thus cannot be relied on to reduce the risk of undetected random error. On days with low patient testing volume, and low numbers of normal patients, the distribution of patient results may be very different than it is in times of normal volume. If there are more outlying patient results, there is more truncation, and the sensitivity of the AoN procedure is probably affected. It is essential to recheck the distribution of patient results periodically. This is especially important for laboratories that test samples from large groups of patients whose care is actively managed toward target laboratory test values. Regular long-term monitoring of monthly patient means and standard deviations would be helpful.

REFERENCES

1. Hoffman RG, Waid NE. The "average of normals" method of quality control. Am J Clin Pathol 1965;43:134–41.
2. Bull BS, Elashoff RM, Heilbron DC, et al. A study of various estimators for the derivation of quality control procedures from patient erythrocyte indices. Am J Clin Pathol 1974;61:473–81.

3. Westgard JO, Cembrowski GS. Relationship of quality goals and measurement performance to the selection of quality control procedures for multi-channel haematology analysers [review]. Eur J Haematol Suppl 1990;53:14–8.
4. Cembrowski GS, Carey RN. Laboratory quality management: QC & QA. Chicago: ASCP Press; 1989.
5. Cembrowski GS, Chandler EP, Westgard JO. Assessment of "average of normal" quality control procedures and guidelines for implementation. Am J Clin Pathol 1984;81:492–7.
6. Westgard JO, Smith FA, Mountain PJ, et al. Design and assessment of average of normal (AON) patient data algorithms to maximize run lengths for automatic process control. Clin Chem 1996;42:1683–8.
7. Westgard JO, Stein B. Automated selection of statistical quality-control procedures to assure meeting clinical or analytical quality requirements. Clin Chem 1997;43: 400–3.
8. Westgard JO. Six sigma quality design and control. Madison (WI): Westgard QC; 2006.
9. Ye JJ, Ingels SD, Parvin CA. Performance evaluation and planning for patient-based quality control procedures. Am J Clin Pathol 2000;113:240–8.

Patient Data Algorithms

Joely A. Straseski, PhD, DABCC*,
Frederick G. Strathmann, PhD, DABCC (CC, TC)

KEYWORDS

- Quality control • Quality assurance • Risk management • Total testing process
- Delta checks • Laboratory errors

KEY POINTS

- Algorithms using individual patient results can be a useful complement to routine quality-control materials.
- Patient results can be used to detect error or identify potential testing complications at all phases of the total testing process (preanalytical, analytical, and postanalytical phases).
- Patient-specific data algorithms include delta checks, tests to verify specimen or tube type, absurdity checks, and result-based reporting.

INTRODUCTION

Quality-control materials are used with every method and on every type of automated analyzer in the modern laboratory. Laboratorians routinely use these types of tools to determine whether an assay is performing adequately. However, quality-control materials alone cannot detect all types of errors or all issues that may arise with a patient specimen. Complementary techniques may be used to address issues beyond the capacity of manufactured control materials. One complementary technique uses patient results to evaluate different aspects of the total testing process, or the preanalytical, analytical, and postanalytical phases of a specimen's lifespan. These results may be assessed on an individual patient level, or among a population. This article focuses on patient data algorithms derived from individual patient results. Population-based algorithms use a different approach and were reviewed elsewhere in this issue by Neill Carey.

Risk is inherent in each step of the total testing process. Deriving specific algorithms based on individual test results is one method that can be used to mitigate these risks. Limitations of traditional quality-control materials include expense, stability, inconsistent matrices, and their inability to assess the specimen quality.[1] In contrast, algorithms specific to individual patient results can aid in determining several issues throughout the total testing process (**Table 1**). They may alert the laboratorian to an

Financial disclosure and conflict of interest: The authors have nothing to disclose.
ARUP Laboratories, University of Utah, 500 Chipeta Way, Mail Code 115, Salt Lake City, UT 84108-1221, USA
* Corresponding author.
E-mail address: joely.a.straseski@aruplab.com

Table 1		
Types of error detection possible throughout the total testing process		
Preanalytical Phase	**Analytical Phase**	**Postanalytical Phase**
Misidentified specimens	Instrumentation errors	True patient changes
Mishandled specimens	Bias	Proper test usefulness
Proper specimen type	Sampling errors	Comparison of POCT and central
Proper specimen collection device		methods

Abbreviation: POCT, point-of-care testing.

analytical issue with the instrumentation used or a possible error in specimen collection. Beyond the laboratory, these types of algorithms can alert health care providers to changes in the patient condition, inadequate specimen type or collection method, or improper test use. However, patient data algorithms and these types of rules may prove difficult to work with. Also, they are not sensitive enough to serve as the sole source of quality management within the laboratory. Because they can detect issues that quality-control materials may not address, they simply provide a complementary tool for assessing and mitigating risk.

This article discusses patient-specific tools that can be used to identify and minimize error at different points throughout the total testing process. These tools are divided into the 3 phases of the testing process: preanalytical, analytical, and postanalytical. Delta checks are the best described of all data algorithms based on results from a single patient. These alerts, which identify serial patient results that differ by more than an allowable amount, are uniquely capable of detecting error throughout the total testing process. Therefore, they are discussed in all three phases. Errors in the preanalytical process can also be interrogated by certain tests to verify both specimen type and proper specimen collection device. The analytical phase has many checks in place in the laboratory, but tools such as delta checks and absurdity checks may also be used. The postanalytical phase again includes delta checks to determine true changes in the patient condition, as well as tests to determine the true usefulness of these checks at the point-of-care (POC) and within the central laboratory, as well as result-based rules for reporting of individual results.

PREANALYTICAL PHASE

The preanalytical phase of the total testing process encompasses many variables and its importance should never be underestimated. As a whole, the phrase "garbage in, garbage out" describes these variables succinctly. Specimen integrity must be ensured if quality results are to be generated. Minimizing risk during this phase can be difficult, if not impossible, for the laboratory to do alone. Risk may be introduced at several steps, including specimen collection, handling, and transportation. Identifying risks before laboratory analysis, or even receipt, is a necessary part of the testing process.

Delta Checks: Preanalytical Phase

Introduction
Delta checks are among the better-described quality tools that use individual patient results. First proposed by Nosanchuk and Gottmann[2] in 1974, Ladenson[3] later fittingly described delta checks as using "patients as their own controls." Delta checks, also referred to as delta limits, failures, or alerts, are the calculated difference between the current patient result and a previous one. If that difference exceeds preestablished limits within a set time interval, an alert or flag is prompted and results are reviewed further.

Delta checks can be caused by either of the following:

Misidentified or mishandled specimen
True biological change in the patient

Identifying fluctuations in patient biology is of paramount concern when evaluating delta check results. Alerting the health care team to relevant deviations from a patient's baseline defines the main purpose of laboratory testing. However, delta checks also play an important role in risk analysis, by identifying excursions from proper sampling practice or handling. Appropriate delta check limits should ideally find a balance between alerting staff to deviations (true-positives) and avoiding unnecessary clinical investigation (false-positives).

Using this type of patient data algorithm, or control, helps identify errors that go beyond what traditional liquid quality-control materials are capable of detecting. Delta checks respond to risks associated with individual patient results, and not only the analytical performance of laboratory methods. They are unique in that they are able to detect issues that may arise at multiple points throughout the total testing process, thus they are discussed in all three phases.

Misidentified or mishandled specimens

Delta checks are capable of identifying numerous preanalytical issues and have an essential role in controlling risk in both the laboratory setting and the patient care environment. These types of preanalytical errors can include, but are not limited to, improper patient identification before sample collection, specimens obtained from or above an intravenous line, use of incorrect anticoagulant or preservative, inappropriate centrifugation speed or duration, unsuitable transport conditions (temperature, ultraviolet exposure, agitation, delayed separation of serum or plasma from cells), or misidentification during laboratory testing (during preparation of aliquots or dilutions). Setting appropriate limits to identify errors helps mitigate risk at each of these preanalytical steps.

Initial reports from the mid-1970s identified manual data entry mistakes as the most common cause of delta check alerts.[3] As laboratory information systems and instrumentation have evolved and become less manual, this statistic has changed. Most delta checks are now associated with true changes in the patient condition or misidentification.[2,4–6] Dufour and colleagues[6] found that 80% of 500 consecutive delta checks were caused by changes in the patient condition. However, the ability of delta check alerts to correctly identify changes in the patient condition is still low. As specimen mix-up error rates go down, delta checks have a decreased ability to detect true changes (positive predictive value). Two separate studies have previously reported predictive values of only 0.4% and 6%.[6,7] More recent studies mimic these findings, with one reporting negligible positive predictive values (<1.4%) at specimen mix-up error rates of less than 1 in 1000, depending on the analyte and delta check equation used.[8] Another study showed mean corpuscular volume to have the highest positive predictive value for specimen mislabeling, out of 11 analytes investigated.[9] The remaining 10 analytes did not exhibit clinical usefulness for identifying mislabeled specimens. Nevertheless, regardless of low predictive values, a large number of delta checks may be used to alert laboratory staff to a possible adverse patient event, thus highlighting their role in managing patient risk and validating their importance.

True biological changes

Delta checks are not always associated with morbidity or mortality. Many changes in the patient condition can lead to significant preanalytical differences in serial laboratory measurements. The cause of these changes can vary from the severe (eg, cardiac or respiratory arrest) to the expected (eg, preprandial vs postprandial glucose), but both delta checks reflect some type of change in the patient condition. They differ only in whether they indicate that medical intervention is warranted. Delta checks may alert the health care team to an unexpected result, possibly one that indicates a pending issue with their patient. It could be argued that providing this type of data to a clinician is the ultimate example of risk management.

Biological, or physiologic, variation is the inherent change that is observed in certain analytes over time and depends on multiple variables. Some sources of biological variation are controllable (diet, physical exertion, posture), whereas others are not (circadian rhythm, menstrual cycle). Common causes of fluctuations in analyte concentration include patient age, inherent differences in patient populations, and recent medical treatments or procedures. Depending on the analyte, biological variation can vary by age, and thus limits that are useful in neonates may not be applicable to an elderly population. In the same way, variation is expected in certain analytes for oncology patients or kidney transplant recipients that are not expected in a healthy adolescent. These inherent differences highlight the importance of setting delta check limits that are appropriate for the patient population. For example, delta checks for creatinine are not useful or appropriate for use in laboratories serving a renal dialysis clinic. Other examples of specific treatments or populations include administration of chemotherapeutic agents or intravenous fluids, feeding tubes, surgery, or organ transplantation. The possibility of variation from these types of sources must be considered when investigating discordant laboratory results.

Candidate analytes

Beyond determining relevance within a patient population (eg, usefulness of creatinine delta checks in patients on dialysis), certain analytes are better candidates than others for setting delta check limits because of their biological actions. To maintain a homeostatic set point within the body, proteins, hormones, and enzymes all attempt to limit overt fluctuations. Some systems are maintained within a tight window (pH, calcium), whereas wider variation is acceptable for others (iron, cholesterol). Delta checks are most appropriate when applied to analytes that vary little from day to day, or those with low intraindividual variation. In these cases, smaller differences between laboratory measurements are needed to identify true changes in analyte concentration. Examples of suitable candidates for applying delta checks include electrolytes, calcium, creatinine, hemoglobin, hematocrit, and mean corpuscular volume. Appropriate risk assessment, or determining the significance of change, requires that each laboratory establishes analyte-specific limits for these candidates, applicable to their patient population.

Two calculations that may be used to identify candidate analytes for delta checks are reference change values (RCV) and the index of individuality (II). Both are described at length by Fraser[10] and Cembrowski and Carey.[1,10] RCVs take both analytical and biological variation into account, determining the amount of change between measurements that would be tolerated if both variables were considered. The RCV is described by the following equation:

$$RCV = 2^{\frac{1}{2}} * Z * \left(CV_A^2 + CV_I^2\right)^{\frac{1}{2}}$$

The Z score is defined as the number of standard deviations appropriate for the probability level and can be defined as bidirectional (both increases and decreases in analyte concentration are relevant) or unidirectional (only an increase or decrease is relevant). At the 95% probability level for a bidirectional analyte, the Z score is 1.96; 99% probability corresponds with a Z score of 2.58. Z-score tables are standard and can be found in most common statistics textbooks. Analytical coefficient of variation (CV_A) describes analytical imprecision, or variation, for the assay and analyte, and is determined from quality-control materials, preferably with a mean near the results being compared or a relevant medical decision point. Intraindividual coefficient of variation (CV_I) refers to the within-subject, or biological, variation expected. These values are often obtained from the literature, from internal studies, or from compiled databases.[11,12] The RCV formula can also be rearranged to solve for Z, which describes the probability that an observed difference between 2 measurements is significant.[10,13,14] Assessing probability addresses risk by ascertaining how much change is acceptable.

The second calculation that provides information relevant to choosing appropriate analytes to monitor via a delta check is the II. First described by Harris[15] in 1974, the II provides a numerical description of how much fluctuation is expected, and relates CV_I to the interindividual (between-subject) coefficient of variation (CV_G).

$$II = CV_I/CV_G$$

When between-subject variation exceeds within-subject variation, the II is low. Low values (<0.6) indicate that an analyte is tightly regulated within an individual, but variation may exist between different people.[16] Analytes with low day-to-day intraindividual variation are desirable candidates for delta checks. In practical terms, a small change in laboratory values for this type of analyte may correspond with a biologically relevant change within the individual. However, the use of reference intervals for these types of measurements is not always useful, because of the large amount of variation between people in a given population. This variation in the population leads to wide reference intervals; thus, small changes observed within an individual may still lie within the reference interval and not be noted as a significant change. Analytes with large II (>1.4) describe the converse of this scenario: delta checks may not be useful, but significant changes may be noted compared with the reference interval.[16] Among other available references, Lacher and colleagues[12] most recently provided a list of II values, along with intraindividual and interindividual variation, for 42 common laboratory analytes using data from the National Health and Nutrition Examination Survey III (NHANES III). Most measured values in the clinical laboratory have a low II, thus calling into question the usefulness of the population-based reference interval and/or delta checks.[17]

Delta checks used for parameters that do not change appreciably within an individual provide a straightforward way of identifying mislabeled or misidentified samples. An example is the disappearance of something that was expected to be present; for example, tumor markers or therapeutic drug values of zero, when appreciable values had previously been measured. Therapeutic drug monitoring, in particular, is not normally requested unless a value is expected. Another example is the comparison of ABO/Rh blood groups or the presence of other antibodies.

Implementation

The most fundamental question to address before implementation of delta check limits is why the laboratory plans to use them. What is the motivation? What types of risk need to be mitigated? If biologically relevant changes are meant to be detected, then the limits must be small and specific to the individual analyte. If detecting misidentified, or inappropriately handled, specimens is the goal, then large limits are appropriate. Tight limits may identify minor changes in the patient condition, but at the risk of flagging false-positive results and initiation of unnecessary and time-consuming investigation. Wide limits minimize these investigations, but increase the risk for false-negatives as well. A balance between both scenarios is key, but is often difficult to obtain. The focus of delta checks can be identified during the initial phases of a risk assessment plan and then implemented accordingly.

Delta checks are defined as a difference in 2 different patient results. The time interval between the two results is also critical to this concept. Which scenario would have greater clinical significance: 2 discrepant results that occurred over a span of 24 hours or over 9 months? As the time span between results increases, it increases the odds that a discrepancy is caused by natural variation or disease progression. Lacher and Connelly[18] incorporated time intervals between collections into their rate check parameter. This is defined as either of the following:

Rate difference = Delta difference/Delta time

Rate percent change = Delta percent change/Delta time

Even when accounting for time intervals, the investigators still concluded that values for hospitalized patients differed from those for ambulatory individuals, reiterating the need for population-specific limits. Another recent approach to assess appropriate time intervals between measurements used time-adjusted sensitivity scores (TAS) to increase the sensitivity and specificity of delta check rules.[19] TAS multiplies sensitivity by repeat ordering frequency for an analyte. Twenty general chemistry analytes were investigated, with results ranging between 1 and 28 days apart. The optimum time interval between analyses for most tests was between 2 and 5 days. The maximum intervals differed by analyte; intervals for enzyme tests were up to 5 days between measurements, electrolyte intervals were much lower, and delta check limits were not effective for analytes such as magnesium and glucose. Determining appropriate usefulness and associated levels of risk is important before implementation of delta check limits, including the appropriate time intervals between measurements.

Once candidate analytes have been selected, establishing delta check limits is traditionally a multifactorial process. Common approaches include using data from population distributions, biological variation, or experience and adjustment over time. Most frequently, a combination of these approaches is used. No single method is capable of identifying all errors, with no false-positives. It is laborious to establish limits empirically based on patient population distributions, but this may be the best way to set limits specific to an institution's patient demographics. The approach is similar to that used to establish a new reference interval. Representative individuals are identified and serial results are gathered. The difference, or delta, between those values is determined and frequencies calculated. Based on the goals of the delta check plan and the initial risk assessment, delta limits can be based on the central 95% or 99% of these results. This method is particularly valuable for unique patient populations, or those that may benefit from identifying and alerting providers to possible changes in the patient condition. There are a handful of studies, most published several years ago, that give examples of biological limits, as obtained from population studies.[3,20,21] Most published limits have been established in healthy populations. Limits are wider in unhealthy subjects, again showing the need for population-specific delta check parameters. Inherent biological variation can also be used to determine delta check limits. RCVs, as described earlier, are often used to determine what constitutes a significant change. Because RCVs account for both analytical and biological variation, all phases of the total testing process are represented (preanalytical, analytical, and postanalytical factors).

The number of ways delta checks can be implemented is only limited by the computer system in place. In addition, limits are analyte dependent. Limits that are commonly used include changes in absolute values, percent change, or a combination of both (eg, absolute values below a certain analyte concentration and percent change at higher concentrations). For some analytes, increases in concentrations within a certain time interval may be more clinically relevant than a decrease (or vice versa). Certain limits may be applied only to certain patient populations, from certain hospital or clinic locations, ordering physicians, and so forth. More complicated limits may first focus on whether a result was within a specified reference interval before triggering further delta check rules. Depending on the analyte, a change from normal to abnormal, or the reverse, may be clinically relevant. Depending on the needs of the laboratory, any of the limits discussed earlier may be used, or a combination of several. A robust laboratory information system and middleware is needed to keep complex rules and combinations in order.

No tables containing examples of delta check limits are provided in this article. This omission is intentional and underscores the importance of establishing and vetting limits within each institution and population.

Specimen Type Verification

Assay performance depends on the type of matrix present in the specimen. Although assay design may be similar among the various matrices approved for use, the calibration is frequently matrix specific and a mismatch between calibrator and specimen matrices can have significant clinical implications. To reduce the potential for patient harm caused by an incorrect calibration-matrix match, a common troubleshooting technique is to assay the specimen for an analyte specific to only 1 of the matrices. For example, if an aliquot of the original specimen is received by the laboratory, a urine specimen may arrive with an order for a serum thyroid-stimulating hormone (TSH). The sample types may look similar, thus the assay would be performed as usual, yielding a suspiciously low TSH concentration. The result may prompt verification of the specimen type by testing total cholesterol. Cholesterol is present in serum, not in urine, therefore suspiciously low cholesterol concentrations may indicate that the wrong specimen type was submitted for testing and further inquiry is warranted. In contrast, a serum specimen may be incorrectly submitted when a urine total protein was ordered. Measuring creatinine can often help resolve the two; urine creatinine values are considerably higher than those found in serum. The result can help direct the laboratory in the interpretation of an unlikely result for urine protein. This simple method of using a known disparity between specimen types for analytes such as cholesterol and creatinine can provide the laboratory with a mechanism to validate a specimen type before an incorrect result is reported.

Tube Type Verification

A subset of laboratory test results from a single specimen can be used in concert to help determine whether a specimen was submitted using an incompatible anticoagulant. A common scenario most often begins with a dangerously increased potassium result for a submitted plasma sample. Before calling a critical, but potentially invalid, potassium result, the calcium and alkaline phosphatase values should be reviewed. A plasma sample that originated from a K_2-ethylenediamine tetraacetic acid (EDTA) tube would result in an extreme increase in potassium (a result of the potassium present in the tube), a substantial reduction in calcium (a result of chelation by EDTA), and a reduction in alkaline phosphatase (a result of magnesium chelation). These 3 laboratory results, when found on a single specimen, can be a strong indicator that further investigation is warranted and may determine whether a potentially incorrect sample type is the reason for the abnormal results. In addition, plasma taken from EDTA-containing blood collection tubes can cause erroneously increased coagulation test results and the potential reporting of invalid critical results. Sodium tetraphenylborate testing has been found to be an effective method to identify samples submitted for coagulation testing in EDTA.[22]

ANALYTICAL PHASE

This phase of the specimen life cycle is defined as the testing of the specimen, and encompasses both manual and automated methods; this is the phase in which laboratorians are often most familiar and comfortable. A large part of their knowledge base is focused on ensuring the optimal performance of the instruments and procedures. The predominant risk associated with this phase of the total testing process is producing an incorrect result. Risk scores could be assigned to describe the most benign outcome to the most severe and possibly life threatening. Traditional quality-control materials are in this category, because they alert technologists to the risk of something going wrong with the testing system as a whole.

Delta Checks: Analytical Phase

Identifying errors in the analytical testing process is the assignment charged to traditional quality-control materials. Because of this internal error detection system, delta checks are not routinely thought of as useful during this phase of specimen testing. However, delta checks are so entwined with all 3 phases of testing that it is easy to identify multiple areas in which delta checks can be used. Setting appropriate delta check limits and reviewing flagged results can significantly reduce the reporting of erroneous results caused by analytical problems.

During the analytical phase of testing, delta checks may reveal either instrument-specific or operator-specific inconsistencies. Identifying a significant difference between serial measurements for a specific analyte may detect instrument-specific issues. Most commonly, observed discrepancies may be caused by different analyzers being used for the 2 different testing events. Laboratories are responsible for verifying comparable performance between identical analyzers at least twice per year,[23] thus true differences would ideally be caught during that process. Delta checks may also recognize sampling issues, such as probe or pipettor inconsistencies including aspiration of inadequate sample volume or the presence of air bubbles. Calibration differences over time may be discovered if delta check alerts routinely flag the second set of results as invariably higher or lower than previous results. Discordance between results that are obtained by 2 different methods or manufacturer's assays may highlight analytical interferences specific to one assay.

A delta check alert may also detect errors in manual procedures or preparation steps. Large variances between results may point out calculation or dilution mistakes, differences in mixing techniques, or errors in other sample handling processes. In the same way, if an assay is subject to variation caused by differences in pH or temperature, a delta check may identify wide variations in these parameters. Large variances between reagent lots may also trigger a delta check alert and prompt further investigation.

Absurdity Checks

Monitoring for laboratory values that deviate excessively from the norm can be an effective method to detect error in all phases of laboratory testing. In the analytical phase, absurdity checks, or implausible values,[24] have been used to uncover problems such as instrument failures, data entry errors, or data transmission problems. Absurdity checks have become a key component in the widespread push for autoverification of laboratory results[25] and form part of the College of American Pathologists requirements for laboratory certification under autoverification.[26] Approaches to detecting spurious laboratory results range from manual review at the bench to statistically guided, decision tree algorithms.[27] Consensus guidelines on what constitutes an absurd value do not exist and citations outlining their use are more than 3 decades old.[20] Statistical tests for outlier detection can be used with questionable effectiveness to provide ranges of unlikely values for absurdity checks,[28] but most laboratories use values determined by the linear range of the assay, clinically relevant limits, or values understood to be inconsistent with life. **Table 2** provides a reference point for establishing of a small number of absurdity values.

Using paired analytes can provide an alternate means for assessing the validity of laboratory results by using natural biological processes, and some logic and mathematics, to dictate rules.[29] For example, several analytes (eg, prostate-specific antigen and thyroid hormones) can be measured and reported as total or free in regards to binding protein association. Situations in which the free fraction is higher than the total fraction could indicate an analytical component that went awry. Total protein concentration similarly should always exceed an albumin value and total bilirubin values should always be higher than the direct bilirubin result. In addition, use of the anion gap is sensitive to errors in ion-selective electrode measurement for sodium, chloride, and bicarbonate when the gap is zero or negative because of the expectation of unmeasured anions in the sample. Any laboratory result that represents a calculation of multiple factors should be checked against each constituent. Errors identified during simple math checks such as these quickly highlight the need for further investigation.

Examples of general biology giving a clue to aberrant results during the analytical phase include either aspartate or alanine aminotransferase being grossly abnormal

Table 2
Examples of absurdity values

Analyte (Serum)	Lower Limit	Upper Limit
mg/dL		
Glucose	50	500
Creatinine	0.3	7.5
Calcium	6.5	13
mmol/L		
Sodium	120	150
Potassium	3	6
Chloride	85	115
Bicarbonate	10	40
U/L		
Alkaline phosphatase	5	250
Creatinine kinase	5	1500

Data from Whitehurst P, Di Silvio TV, Boyadjian G. Evaluation of discrepancies in patients' results–an aspect of computer-assisted quality control. Clin Chem 1975;21(1):87–92.

on its own; both enzymes traditionally follow each other during hepatic injury or disease. Hemoglobin and hematocrit or creatinine and urea nitrogen concentrations also customarily mirror each other. Feedback loops provide another means for verification; in normal situations, increased TSH values cause increases in free thyroxine as well. Disease processes can alter these loops and cause unexpected results, but confirming whether these types of results are expected within the context of the clinical picture is another step in the process to minimize risk. Therefore, similar to delta checks, consideration of the patient population is critical when determining the usefulness of these types of parallel checks.

POSTANALYTICAL PHASE

During the final portion of the total testing process, patient data algorithms continue to aid in the minimization of risk and help to ensure that high-quality, accurate results are being produced. Even after results have been generated, the results can be part of the quality process.

Delta Checks: Postanalytical Phase

Most importantly, delta checks need to be used in concert with the biological picture with which the patient has presented. Correlation between laboratory results and patient condition is key to proper patient care. Without this essential step, laboratory tests cannot be correctly interpreted and are not useful in the context of the patient as a whole. Delta checks may alert a health care provider to a clinical situation of which they were unaware, and may illicit further questioning of an unexpected result. Within this context, delta checks serve as a risk moderator if clinicians are alerted to something that was not originally their focus.

Similar to the tests of biology and mathematics that were described earlier, another test of logic can be applied once several results have been generated and studied. If delta check alerts have been flagged for multiple analytes for a particular patient, this increases the chance that a preanalytical error has occurred. If one delta check alert has been flagged, but the delta (difference) is exaggerated (eg, greater than 3 times the existing delta limit for that analyte), this also increases the likelihood that patient identification or another preanalytical specimen collection procedure has been compromised.

Delta Check Utilization in Point-of-care Testing

Modern delta check calculations make use of the laboratory information system or middleware software program, substantially reducing the impact on workflow and allowing an increased number and potential complexity of delta check rules. Although routinely used in the central laboratory, delta checks in the POC environment can prove difficult. POC testing often lacks access to centralized data and limits the operator's ability to have statistical analyses applied to patient results in real time.[30] Rapid-testing (STAT) labs or point-of-service laboratories have provided a potentially successful compromise between obtaining the right test in the needed time frame and allowing the use of the laboratory software for delta check calculations.[31]

Despite these common limitations in the information technology infrastructure, delta checks can be used to compare results between POC and centralized laboratory methods. POC methods inherently contain risk, commonly because of imprecision issues, thus minimizing those risks is critical. Considerable differences in methodology and sample type preclude the use of stringent comparison criteria, thus these comparisons are often informal ones. Different rules or limits may be used by the two methods, but a comparison between them may still be useful. For example, widely disparate differences between POC and automated glucose results may indicate an interference (eg, documented maltose interference with glucose dehydrogenase pyrro-loquinoline quinone testing strips) or issue with sampling (eg, improperly cleaned fingertip) that affects one result and not the other. In the case of glucose, the decision whether to administer insulin would be different depending on which result was obtained first.

Evaluation of Delta Check Usefulness

Delta checks may be applied in a variety of ways, each specific to the type of detection desired by the laboratory. Once delta checks or any other measure of risk mitigation are instituted, follow-up is needed to determine whether these metrics are working adequately and alerting staff to the issues they are meant to detect. Few metrics exist to determine usefulness; however, usefulness of newly implemented alerts can be assessed in a manner similar to determining the clinical usefulness of laboratory tests (namely, sensitivity and specificity determinations). Sensitivity and specificity measures can be applied to describe the accuracy of the chosen alerts. As mentioned earlier, delta checks can be used to detect specific types of error that affect those areas on which the laboratory chooses to focus (eg, mislabeled specimens, biological changes in the patient). In the context of delta checks, sensitivity refers to the ability of a limit or rule to accurately detect a sample that is affected by the specific issue the laboratory wants to detect. Specificity describes the opposite scenario: whether the delta limit correctly omits those specimens that are error free. These two metrics have been used by some recent computer modeling studies to determine the usefulness of delta checks.

Automated mislabel detection represents one of many applications for delta check calculations. Delta check calculations have been routinely adopted in many laborato-ries with automated systems and their use is indicated in the general checklist of the College of American Pathologists, GEN.43890.[26] Mislabel detection using delta checks is a common practice, but 2 recent articles have described their limitations. In 2011, Strathmann and colleagues[9] used a simulation study to show the ineffective-ness of absolute delta calculations to detect mislabeled specimens at several mislabel rates. Several commonly used analytes were assessed for their usefulness in delta check calculations with distributions for calculated deltas compared between correctly labeled and mislabeled pairs. A summary table was provided that showed the effect of varying the delta check cutoffs on sensitivity, specificity, and positive predictive value at mislabel rates of 1 in 500, 1 in 1000, and 1 in 5000. The investigators concluded that the total number of delta failures was most sensitive to the cutoff value used rather than the prevalence of mislabels; delta checks were useful for detecting mislabels only when the error rate was extremely high. This finding is consistent with the notion that most failed deltas are false-positives in the context of mislabel identification. In addition, the investigators' results from 2 institutions with nearly iden-tical automated chemistry and hematology platforms showed that a common cut-and-paste approach to delta cutoff establishment from one institution to another when patient populations are not comparable is invalid and should not be done. A second article in 2012 reported similar conclusions and added further evidence for the limited usefulness of using delta checks for mislabel detection.[8]

Result-based Rules for Reporting

As mentioned earlier, correlating current results against other related values can iden-tify errors that may have occurred at previous points in the total testing process. Absur-dity checks are one example. A patient result can also serve as a decision point for

Table 3
Examples of result-based rules for reporting

Analyte	Rule Summary
Rules Based on Specimen Integrity:	
Potassium	When serum or plasma potassium is performed and the result is within analytical measuring range and hemolysis index is greater than 150 mg/dL, include the following comment: "This specimen is hemolyzed. This may cause the potassium result to be falsely increased."
Urine concentration	When 24-h urine creatinine is performed and the result is less than 25 mg/dL, include the following comment: "Specimens containing less than 25 mg/dL creatinine may be too dilute for reliable testing."
Rules Based on Patient Demographics:	
Estradiol	When serum or plasma estradiol is performed by immunoassay and the result is less than 20 pg/mL, and the patient is female >18 y old, include the following comment: "Estradiol result is low by immunoassay. Suggest repeat testing with more sensitive method."
LDL-chol	When LDL calculation is performed by Freidwald equation and triglyceride concentration is greater than or equal to 400 mg/dL, include the following comment: "LDL-chol value cannot be calculated because of increased triglycerides. Triglycerides greater than 400 mg/dL interfere with LDL calculations."

Abbreviation: LDL-chol, low-density lipoprotein cholesterol.

several checks that can be performed before sending those results to the patient chart. These types of checks may be referred to as discern rules (**Table 3**). Based on the patient result, and perhaps additional demographic information, result-based reporting rules may provide guidance for optimal patient care and/or proper laboratory test use. For example, a 1,25-dihydroxyvitamin D result may prompt an accompanying comment directing the clinician to order 25-hydroxyvitamin D testing if assessment of traditional vitamin D stores is desired. Testosterone results determined by immunoassay methods may similarly be automatically checked against patient age and gender. If the immunoassay result was requested for a woman or child, that result may prompt a comment indicating that mass spectrometry has increased sensitivity at lower testosterone concentrations and is the preferred testing method in patients in whom low values are expected. These types of reporting rules can also be used as a guide to physicians in situations in which recommended testing is unclear, such as adding comments to chromium and cobalt joint fluid test results that suggest serum as the preferred method for assessing failure of metal-on-metal prosthetic devices. Providing this type of additional comment alerting clinicians to a specific reporting situation may mitigate the risk of reporting erroneous results or results for the wrong patient and may provide a medium to educate and update physicians on test use.

SUMMARY

Certain amounts of risk are inherent to every part of the total testing process, from patient preparation and sample collection to reporting of results. Testing algorithms that use individual patient results can be a useful means to perform quality checks throughout this process. The types of checks described in this article complement traditional laboratory quality-control processes; neither patient-derived checks nor routine quality-control materials are capable of detecting all types of error.

The methods discussed here should not be applied in a cut-and-paste format, because one size does not fit all when it comes to patient-derived data algorithms. The patient population must be carefully considered when rules and limits are being implemented. When used properly, patient results can become a useful component of the quality-control toolbox that works to minimize risk and increase the quality of individual patient results.

REFERENCES

1. Cembrowski GS, Carey RN. Laboratory quality management: QC and QA. Chicago: ASCP; 1989.
2. Nosanchuk JS, Gottmann AW. CUMS and delta checks. A systematic approach to quality control. Am J Clin Pathol 1974;62(5):707–12.
3. Ladenson JH. Patients as their own controls: use of the computer to identify "laboratory error". Clin Chem 1975;21(11):1648–53.
4. Sher PP. An evaluation of the detection capacity of a computer-assisted real-time delta check system. Clin Chem 1979;25(6):870–2.
5. Iizuka Y, Kume H, Kitamura M. Multivariate delta check method for detecting specimen mix-up. Clin Chem 1982;28(11):2244–8.
6. Dufour DR, Cruser DL, Buttolph T, et al. The clinical significance of delta checks. Am J Clin Pathol 1998;110:531.
7. Kim JW, Kim JQ, Kim SI. Differential application of rate and delta check on selected clinical chemistry tests. J Korean Med Sci 1990;5(4):189–95.
8. Ovens K, Naugler C. How useful are delta checks in the 21 century? A stochastic-dynamic model of specimen mix-up and detection. J Pathol Inform 2012;3:5.
9. Strathmann FG, Baird GS, Hoffman NG. Simulations of delta check rule performance to detect specimen mislabeling using historical laboratory data. Clin Chim Acta 2011;412(21–22):1973–7.
10. Fraser CG. Biological variation: from principles to practice. Washington, DC: AACC; 2001.
11. Ricos C, Alvarez V, Cava F, et al. Current databases on biologic variation: pros, cons and progress. Scand J Clin Lab Invest 1999;59:491–500, 2012 update. Available at: http://www.westgard.com/biodatabase1.htm. Accessed October 8, 2012.
12. Lacher DA, Hughes JP, Carroll MD. Estimate of biological variation of laboratory analytes based on the third national health and nutrition examination survey. Clin Chem 2005;51(2):450–2.
13. Katzmann JA, Snyder MR, Rajkumar SV, et al. Long-term biological variation of serum protein electrophoresis M-spike, urine M-spike, and monoclonal serum free light chain quantification: implications for monitoring monoclonal gammopathies. Clin Chem 2011;57(12):1687–92.
14. Cheuvront SN, Fraser CG, Kenefick RW, et al. Reference change values for monitoring dehydration. Clin Chem Lab Med 2011;49(6):1033–7.
15. Harris EK. Effects of intra- and interindividual variation on the appropriate use of normal ranges. Clin Chem 1974;20(12):1535–42.
16. Harris EK. Statistical aspects of reference values in clinical pathology. Prog Clin Pathol 1981;8:45–66.
17. Ceriotti F, Hinzmann R, Panteghini M. Reference intervals: the way forward. Ann Clin Biochem 2009;46(Pt 1):8–17.
18. Lacher DA, Connelly DP. Rate and delta checks compared for selected chemistry tests. Clin Chem 1988;34(10):1966–70.

19. Sampson ML, Rehak NN, Sokoll LJ, et al. Time adjusted sensitivity analysis: a new statistical test for the optimization of delta check rules. J Clin Ligand Assay 2007;30(1–2):44–54.
20. Whitehurst P, Di Silvio TV, Boyadjian G. Evaluation of discrepancies in patients' results–an aspect of computer-assisted quality control. Clin Chem 1975;21(1): 87–92.
21. Wheeler LA, Sheiner LB. Delta check tables for the Technicon SMA 6 continuous-flow analyzer. Clin Chem 1977;23(2 Pt 1):216–9.
22. Crist RA, Gibbs K, Rodgers GM, et al. Effects of EDTA on routine and specialized coagulation testing and an easy method to distinguish EDTA-treated from citrated plasma samples. Lab Hematol 2009;15(4):45–8.
23. CLSI. Verification of comparability of patient results within one health care system; approved guideline, in CLSI Document C54-A-IR. Wayne (PA): Clinical Laboratory Standards Institute; 2012.
24. CLSI. Laboratory quality control based on risk management; approved guideline, in CLSI Document EP23-A. Wayne (PA): Clinical and Laboratory Standards Institute; 2011.
25. Crolla LJ, Westgard JO. Evaluation of rule-based autoverification protocols. Clin Leadersh Manag Rev 2003;17(5):268–72.
26. College of American Pathologists, CAP. Accreditation program. Northfield (IL): College of American Pathologists; 2012.
27. Baron JM, Mermel CH, Lewandrowski KB, et al. Detection of preanalytic laboratory testing errors using a statistically guided protocol. Am J Clin Pathol 2012; 138(3):406–13.
28. Leen, TK, Erdogmus D, Kazmierczak S. Statistical error detection for clinical laboratory tests, in IEEE Engineering in Medicine and Biology Conference. San Diego, August 28–September 1, 2012.
29. Lacher DA. Relationship between delta checks for selected chemistry tests. Clin Chem 1990;36(12):2134–6.
30. Jones BA, Meier FA. Patient safety in point-of-care testing. Clin Lab Med 2004; 24(4):997–1022.
31. Paxton A. Moving the sicker quicker with ER point-of-care. CAP Today 2004;60.

A Strategic Informatics Approach to Autoverification

Jay B. Jones, PhD, DABCC

KEYWORDS

- Autoverification • Informatics • Middleware • Connectivity • Sigma analysis
- Information systems

KEY POINTS

- New informatics tools such as middleware, wide area networks, and virtual servers are enabling a multi-site enterprise approach to lab testing autoverification.
- Autoverification should be planned strategically keeping in mind new developments such as instrument generated orders, increasing interoperability with other information systems, and reflexive testing.
- A quality control plan should be written to include autoverification and its likely evolution in the future.
- Parameters for autoverification should be tabulated in spreadsheets so they may be easily changed and maintained.

INTRODUCTION

Autoverification is frequently described in terms of efficiency gain, cost reduction, and a means of increasing productivity. Alternatively, autoverification may be described as a means to assure quality. A classic approach to autoverification has typically included the generation of decision rules, including those of specimen-based quality control (QC), to rule out or except individual specimens or specimen results that may be suspect or erroneous and automatically verify the rest.[1] Indeed, the foundation of autoverification is the classic QC that has been practiced by laboratories for decades. QC, however, is a very broad term and has evolved well beyond simply testing control material that mimics patient specimens to judge statistical accuracy and precision. QC has come to include error detection, patient information verification, specimen quality judgment, and timeliness of result reporting, to name a few components. Inherent to quality are practices that generate metrics. Quality is proven statistically not just practiced operationally. Superimposed on this expanding definition of quality is the use of modern informatics and automation tools. Hence, it is important to combine and

The author has nothing to disclose.
Division of Laboratory Medicine 01-31, Geisinger Medical Center, Geisinger Health System, 100 North Academy Avenue, Danville, PA 17822-0131, USA
E-mail address: JbuJones@Geisinger.edu

Clin Lab Med 33 (2013) 161–181
http://dx.doi.org/10.1016/j.cll.2012.11.004
0272-2712/13/$ – see front matter © 2013 Elsevier Inc. All rights reserved.

labmed.theclinics.com

update all of the concepts and components of quality to generate new QC plans. To develop such a QC plan, one must first understand where modern QC must be embedded: in laboratory informatics systems.

AUTOVERIFICATION AND EXPANDING LABORATORY INFORMATICS

Basic rule sets for autoverification have not significantly changed for most laboratories and laboratory information systems (LIS) for the past 20 years. With increasing use of newer informatics tools and general expansion of networks, client servers, and middleware, new capabilities for autoverification have become universally available. One must now think in more global terms; verified test results exist in a large continuum of which the LIS is but one part. Coupled with a more global explosion of health information technology (HIT), these new tools are becoming not just focused at the laboratory workstation level but are also being integrated into the mainstream of information flow of the enterprise.[2] It is important for laboratorians to understand how this rapid expansion of health care informatics will impact the laboratory where it provides a very basic informatics component, the laboratory test result, to overall medical decision support in patient care. Laboratory strategy needs to open up to this much larger realm of real-time decision support and not be confined by a factory mentality focusing at just a single workstation verifying or autoverifying a single result.[3]

Wide area networks (WAN) have become ubiquitous in the health care environment. Their presence has enabled real-time interoperability between various entities and information systems in the health care enterprise both functionally and geographically. The laboratory should not be considered a geographic entity within preset walls; rather, it should be viewed as an analytical enterprise spread to wherever laboratory medicine is practiced across a heath care system with information shared at the speed of light. This more global view of the laboratory represents today's reality and will even more significantly become part of the laboratory's future. As interoperable health care informatics continues to be rolled out, extremely powerful tools will present to the laboratory in terms of not just the WAN but also rows of virtual client servers supporting new laboratory applications housed in highly secure and efficient data centers. Virtual client servers housed in data centers is already a predominant model in health care.

Autoverification, again, will be an important strategy to adopt in the future as information flows through this mainstream of health care informatics in an increasingly real-time manner. Paramount in this increasingly global automated flow of real-time information will be the maintenance of statistically defined quality.[4] Poor quality must not be automated. A strategic approach must be taken that defines and preserves quality as the momentum for rolling out increasingly automated health care systems accelerates. It is important to be strategically proactive now to keep up with the pace of accelerating change. One must adapt by creating a QC plan.

DEVELOPING A QC PLAN

Planning and proper documentation is important in expanding classic QC practice into an enterprise autoverification system. Classic QC practices may be envisioned as building blocks in the foundation of this plan. They must be planned to remain integral to the overall structure but rearranged and integrated into modern information systems. Autoverification parameters that should be embedded in the QC plan, which are discussed individually, are shown in **Box 1**.

The key long-term strategy remains how to effectively roll out the QC plan to information systems over time. In the Geisinger Health System, this rollout occurred incrementally over approximately 10 years as the system at large automated to an

Box 1
Components of autoverification to include in a QC plan
Delta checks
Verification limits
Serum indices
Boolean rules (middleware)
Automated QC

electronic medical record and required sharing common information systems for admission/discharge/transfer (A/D/T) and billing. This information technology (IT) framework greatly influences the laboratory's strategic QC plan; therefore, a description of the Geisinger information systems environment is necessary.

Management aspects of creating a QC plan would be expected to vary greatly between health care systems. Vetting of plans by groups and individuals is necessary. Maintaining versionized spreadsheets of individual parameters is important because they form the basis for information system input and change management. Abiding by rules established by the information systems department is mandatory in the era of systems security. There are many factors that influence the timeliness and efficiency of creating and executing the QC plan. The structure of enterprise autoverification in the Geisinger system demonstrates one QC plan that is in advanced stages of development. It is hoped that as a prototype, it may help others strategically plan their own QC plan.

OVERVIEW OF ENTERPRISE ANALYTICS IN THE GEISINGER HEALTH SYSTEM

Examples of an enterprise approach to laboratory quality exist not only in large systems, such as the Geisinger Health System, but also in smaller-scale local community hospitals that have local outreach to community physicians and patients. Just as point-of-care testing is reaching out to patient care and local physicians on a more real-time enterprise basis, autoverified central laboratory testing will do the same. Again, taking a more global approach, one must view the overall process that preserves the preanalytical quality of test/specimen order that is also autoverified with computerized physician order entry (CPOE). The global enterprise strategy[5] must take into account the order process as well as the resulting process. Test result quality must consist of preventing both garbage in (autoverification of CPOE) as well as garbage out (autoverification of test results).

The strategic view of autoverification must also include robust documentation of policy to prevent automation of poor quality.[6–8] With a large system such as the Geisinger Health System, with 70 testing locations on a WAN, having as much standardized and centralized as possible helps alleviate the burden of documenting quality and policy. Using a common collective enterprise approach to laboratory ordering and laboratory resulting with best practice quality allows for a more standard approach for documenting and maintaining quality. The more global HIT approach of the enterprise facilitates laboratory use of document control systems and other quality systems to embed in its own process. The Geisinger system for example, uses a universally accessible document control system on its WAN-based INFOweb called Site Executive (Systems Alliance Inc., Hunt Valley, Maryland) to document laboratory quality policies, laboratory methods, and other important documents to establish best quality practice. This documentation is universally available on the intranet WAN to all providers in the system and may be accessed even from home. Included in this documentation is policy and parameters for autoverification of laboratory tests, no matter where they are performed within the enterprise.

The enterprise approach and future strategy for implementation of laboratory policy must include preanalytical as well as analytical error detection[9] and a means to constantly improve the overall process. One must not approach autoverification as a once-and-done project that gets completed and stays completed. As hardware and software tool sets improve, so must autoverification improve in terms of efficiency and quantifiable quality outcomes. Ongoing improvement of autoverification must also factor in that it will be rapidly expanded in the future to include real-time decision support. A proactive strategic approach should include the prediction of expansion areas, including hardware and increasing clinical demands, to keep up with the accelerated pace of expansion and change.

There are significant burdens to maintaining autoverification. A strategic approach should take into account the impact of ongoing maintenance in sustaining and expanding autoverification. Regulations will continue to impact with requirements[10] to test autoverification protocols whenever significant changes occur. For example with software version upgrades, retesting should be performed. Autoverification components not just in the LIS but also those found in middleware should be critically examined from a maintenance standpoint.[11] Because middleware software exists more on the laboratory side of the operation as opposed to part of the typical LIS environment, the burden rests with laboratorians to perform maintenance and testing. Most laboratorians do not fully appreciate how extensive this maintenance chore may be.

In many cases, the middleware component also serves as a vital interface engine between all enterprise instruments and LIS on a WAN and may be viewed as a single point of failure. Middleware, therefore, becomes a critical testing component for laboratory information flow and needs to be maintained, tested, and deemed safe from a security standpoint.

There is much to consider in developing a long-term strategic plan for autoverification.[11] All components will not be implemented at the same time, and the rollout of autoverification will not be a once-and-done proposition. It is important to start somewhere and get on with it, trusting that over time a strategic plan will improve autoverification and its integration into laboratory IT as it evolves.

The future is very bright in terms of enhanced autoverification. As part of the strategic plan, one needs to also factor in operational considerations and help drive autoverification enhancement with a return on investment in personnel savings as personnel become less available to laboratories. Much has been written about saving cost and increasing productivity with autoverification[12,13]; but in the future, this may evolve to be more of a survival strategy as development time and personnel resources become scarcer.

As autoverification allows us to survive the medical technologist shortage, we will also be confronted with increasing expectations for what is best termed *real-time front-end decision support*. Instruments that are decentralized on a WAN in locations such as emergency and operating rooms may be viewed as centralized laboratory satellite instruments and, as such, managed by stat laboratories rather than point-of-care testing (POCT) coordinators. These instruments, similar to point-of-care instruments, may be viewed as having real-time orders placed and uploaded (ie, autoverified) to the LIS as an instrument-generated order (IGO). Hence, autoverification will become even more extensive in automating both the order and result in POCT and satellite instruments with only ex post facto result review.

Much of this new genre of decentralized testing has already been predicted by industry with new instruments that are placed in point-of-care areas that integrate into a stat laboratory environment. Industry recognizes the need for the modernization of interface standards to support much more interoperability of this genre of testing.[14] An organization has recently been created that has made rapid progress toward replacing older instrument interface standards, such as the American Standards for Testing and Materials 31.14[15] (now Clinical Laboratory Standards Institute LIS 1 and 2),[16] with newer Health Level 7 (HL7) interface specifications. The Industrial In Vitro Diagnostics Connectivity Consortium (IICC, www.IVDconnectivity.org), working within the framework of another standards development organization, Integrating the Health care Enterprise (IHE, http://www.iheusa.org/index.aspx), has recently successfully completed a connect-a-thon. Several IICC member instrument vendors showed at this event that updated instrument interface standards work seamlessly in an interoperable environment.

Hence, many strategic factors must be taken into account when envisioning current as well as future expanded autoverification as instruments and clinical processes become more integrated and automated.[17] Details and examples are presented in the following sections, showing how these strategic factors have been considered and addressed in the Geisinger Health System with their progressive HIT systems.

AN ENTERPRISE APPROACH TO AUTOVERIFICATION

It is important to design autoverification from an information systems standpoint to fit into the mainstream of the information flow of the enterprise.[18] The Geisinger Health System has a well-developed enterprise health care system on a WAN as shown in **Fig. 1**. The WAN connects an electronic health record (EHR) (Epicare, Madison, Wisconsin) throughout all its various entities and, as such, is the ubiquitous CPOE system for the laboratory. Upwards of 10 000 Epicare workstations throughout the enterprise may order tests through CPOE and pass these orders to the LIS (Sunquest, Phoenix, Arizona). Results are shared among providers and patients alike either through the Epic system behind a security firewall on the WAN or a patient Web portal called MyGeisinger outside of the security firewall. More than 200 000 patients have access to laboratory results from their home via an Internet browser. It is, therefore, important to realize that as laboratories anywhere in the system automatically verify laboratory results, they populate not just Epicare for provider review but are sent on for patient review within 48 hours. The distribution of laboratory results is largely an automated system; so as previously mentioned, one must envision the global evolution of automation and passing of results to various stages and levels of review once verified.

As shown in **Fig. 2**, within the Geisinger laboratory departmental enterprise system, chemistry instruments from all locations on the WAN interface via the Data Innovation (DI) Instrument Manager (Data Innovations, Burlington, Vermont) version 8.10 middleware product on a virtual server in the Geisinger Data Center.[19] In turn, DI serves as an interface engine to send all test results to the Sunquest LIS and a BioRad (Hercules, California) virtual server running the QC software, Unity Real Time (URT). The chemistry instrument platforms are highly standardized not just in vendor type but also in technical configuration and reagent use. Single lot numbers of unassayed chemistry QC serum (BioRad Liquichek levels 1, 2) and serum calibrator (Roche CFAS [Roche Diagnostics, Indianapolis, Indiana]) are used for general chemistry at all Geisinger practice sites with instrumentation. All of these instruments are interfaced with common test codes populating the LIS archive no matter where the testing is performed. Reference ranges, methodology, procedure manuals, technical information for providers in a service directory, turnaround time standards, analytical measurement ranges, comment codes, and specimen requirements are all held in common across the system as much as technically feasible. Standardization has been

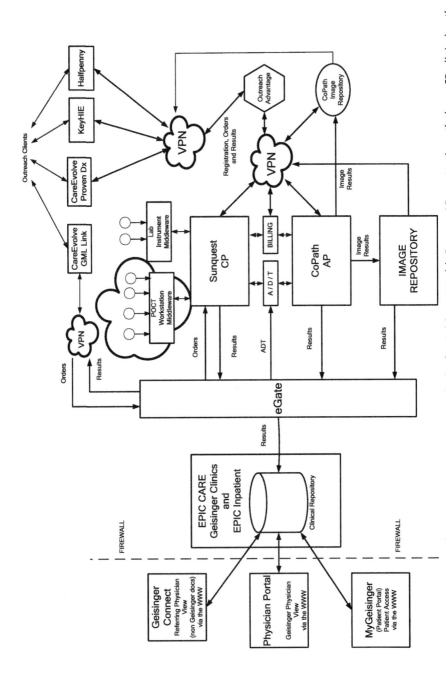

Fig. 1. The laboratory results interface and enterprise connectivity in the Geisinger Health System. AP, anatomic pathology; CP, clinical pathology; eGate, electronic gate interface engine; GML link, Geisinger medical laboratory link; KeyHIE, Key Stone Health Information Exchange; proven Dx, proven diagnostics; VPN, virtual private network; www, World Wide Web.

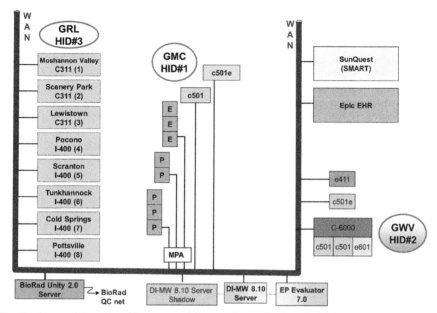

Fig. 2. Connectivity of rapid response laboratories and 2 hospital laboratories via a WAN and shared systems of data innovations middleware (DI-MW) server, BioRad Unity QC software server, Sunquest LIS, and Epicare electronic health record (EHR). GRL, Geisinger regional laboratories; GMC, Geisinger Medical Center; GWV, Geisinger Wyoming Valley; HID, hospital identifier for Sunquest LIS; MPA, Modular Pre analytics.

approached to be both broad and deep in the last decade and a half. Technical depth is reflected in recognition by the College of American Pathologists (CAP) for system accreditation of all affiliated hospital and rapid response laboratories shown in **Fig. 2**. This enterprise analytics strategic approach has proven extremely efficient in reducing redundancy and complexity for laboratory informatics.

Because there is this common and standardized hardware pathway for verifying standardized tests to a single LIS, autoverification parameters have also been standardized. A basic set of autoverification rules has been established to support the enterprise analytical system in chemistry. A similar approach has been taken in hematology using Sysmex Work Area Manager (Sysmex America, Lincolnshire, Illinois) middleware and standardized instrumentation across the Geisinger enterprise. POCT is a third major area whereby hundreds of POCT devices share a common TELCOR (Lincoln, Nebraska) middleware workstation for resulting into Sunquest.

Standardized autoverification parameters include assigned verify limits, in most cases, for the various chemistry platforms running harmonized reagent systems. These verify limits are built into Sunquest LIS tables and, hence, are the focus of autoverification creation and maintenance. Likewise, delta checks have been established in the LIS for the enterprise. QC results and serum indices are captured and archived by DI middleware as interfaced results flow to Sunquest; however, the source of truth for autoverification is Sunquest. Hence, QC results and serum index results populate files in Sunquest, within the limits of Sunquest autoverification functionality. QC results are stored in Sunquest in a very classic fashion because Sunquest is a legacy LIS and serum indices are filed as an instrument message rather than an actual absorbance value. Autoverification in the LIS is, hence, triggered by rules and tables that are built (and importantly maintained) in the LIS even though most raw data are archived in DI middleware.

Even though the source of truth for QC and serum indices resides in the LIS where verification is formalized, identical QC and serum index results are archived in DI and serve an important accessory role in judging quality. A second virtual server in the data center, running Biorad URT QC software, extracts and archives QC point data from DI. It is extremely important to understand the value of data flow in these sorts of accessory systems to establish rules for autoverification. The QC archive in Biorad URT is used as a means to accumulate and tabulate system QC data for specific lot numbers and test methods. The actual statistical peer comparisons are performed on scheduled days; standard deviation intervals (SDI) and coefficient of variation, relative (CVR) are returned from an outside BioRad QC Net server. One has these statistical QC data to base QC performance and autoverification rules on. The Unity real-time peer-compared reports returned by the QC Net server are condensed in several statistical and graphic formats so judgment of bias and imprecision is easy to spot. The process is very automated once established and, hence, more likely to be adequately reviewed. Reams of paper that can be printed in this rich statistical comparison are now replaced by a PDF file, which can easily be stored on network drives after an electronic signature of review. Affiliate reports may also be generated from internally designated laboratory testing sites as a means to cross compare internally generated data.

Similarly, serum index absorbance data for every test done on every instrument in the enterprise are archived within the DI database. These data may then be extracted from DI via an online database connectivity (ODBC) protocol supported by DI. Data may be extracted to Microsoft (MS, Redmond, Washington) Excel or MS Access database programs for further analysis. This information is valuable for examining preanalytical specimen quality across the enterprise. If structured so that serum indices may be associated by location or even by phlebotomist, valuable information may be generated for patterns of hemolysis, lipemia, or icterus across the system. One may use this information to create evidence for establishing rejection rules on serum indices by test to be structured within LIS autoverification. **Fig. 3** shows a survey of serum hemolytic indices over a 3-day period for the system. The histogram from an MS Excel template statistics program shows most specimens are far less than any rejection criteria for hemolysis. However, the tail of a few hemolyzed specimens go to higher levels whereby, in this example, 0.8% of specimens would fail a hemolysis rejection criteria of 130. One can judge the rejection rate by test with this sort of information. Statistics also relate this failure level to a sigma statistic, which again is valuable parametric evidence for making rejection decisions in autoverification.

A formalized effort has been created to standardize statistical QC analysis in the Geisinger system and embed it into autoverification criteria. All chemistry analyzers shown in **Fig. 2** use the same calibration lot number and QC lot number across the system. Hence, comparable data are generated during the QC process at all of the sites and may be collected from the common data archive of the DI middleware. After being sent to BioRad for peer comparison and statistical summarization, these QC data are then further reviewed on an individual site basis as well as on an enterprise basis. Problems in QC performance are assessed by site and test. It is often helpful to troubleshoot a problem test online at a given site by cross comparing URT Levy-Jennings multilevel charts, which are available real time at each laboratory site.

ENTERPRISE SIGMA ANALYSIS

Besides the statistical analysis of individual site QC data,[20] there is a new horizon in applying QC on an enterprise basis with multisite laboratory systems. Using a module within the URT software, called Westgard Advisor (BioRad Laboratories, Hercules,

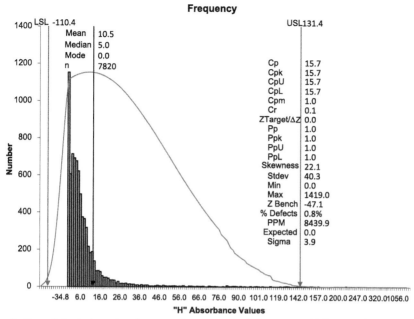

Fig. 3. Hemolytic index absorbance values extracted from DI middleware for Geisinger Health System (all chemistry instruments) over 3-day period.

California), one may create sigma statistics on a monthly basis from peer-compared means (SDIs), CVRs, and total allowable error (TEa). The sigma statistic from West-gard Advisor is calculated for each Geisinger laboratory site and placed in a spread-sheet, which has become a sigma dashboard for the enterprise analytical system.[21] An example for serum potassium is given in **Fig. 4**. Although there is some variation of monthly sigma monitored within a given site and among the various Geisinger sites, several tests remain remarkably stable in terms of ongoing monthly sigma trend. Several tests have been found over the last year to generate consistent monthly sigmas far more than 4 to allow for choosing less stringent Westgard rules for daily QC. Especially enzymes with total allowable error as defined in Clinical Laboratory Improvement Amendment (CLIA) standards of 20% to 30% have proven to have sigmas comfortably more than 6. In those cases, using OPSpecs charts,[22] the auto-verification QC rules have been opened from 1-2s to 1-3s and false rejection rates have dramatically declined by approximately 75%. During this period, there have not been increased failures of CAP proficiency testing or significant downward trends on the monthly sigma dashboard monitors. The author's institution has not yet quan-titated the time savings generated by doing 75% fewer rejections of high-volume chemistry tests, but the overall judgment is that it has decreased distraction and disruption with QC reruns at very busy automated chemistry workstations. One must realize that these disruptions and distractions do not only require unnecessary repeats of QC but also disrupt autoverification. It may take several minutes or even an hour to recover from a QC failure depending on workload. During this recovery period, as it disables autoverification, QC repeat holds up verification of normal patient results. Hence, the autoverification rate should be judged not just by how many spec-imens on a percentage basis qualify for autoverification but also by what percentage of time is the analytical system autoverifying. If there are frequent disruptions to

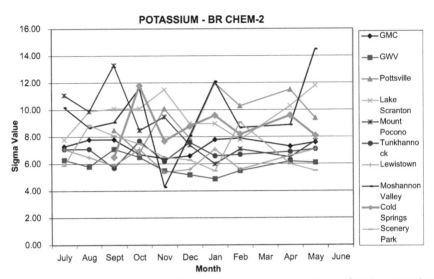

Fig. 4. Monthly sigma dashboard for Geisinger chemistry laboratories performing potassium testing with BioRad level 2 serum QC material. BR CHEM-2, BioRad Chemistry level 2 control; GMC, Geisinger Medical Center; GWV, Geisinger Wyoming Valley.

autoverification, even though the autoverification rate may be 80%, the functional autoverification rate may be 50% and patient results that may have normally been autoverified will be delayed.

The successful implementation of a sigma dashboard monitoring system to chemistry has encouraged the examination of a similar system for hematology and coagulation. For example, hemoglobin as part of a hematology panel has TEa as defined by CLIA as 7%. Typical comparison of the means and coefficients of variation to hematology peer data has generated typical sigmas of 10 for hemoglobin; hence, the author's institution is in the process of abandoning 1-2s rules for hemoglobin and replacing them with 1-3S rules for autoverification at enterprise sites.

In summary, autoverification needs to be incorporated into a much broader enterprise system with electronic connectivity to multiple systems and subsystems to produce efficiency and reduce the possibility of error. The overhead to maintain this broad system will be greatly minimized, especially in multi-entity health systems if properly strategized and designed.

PROFICIENCY TESTING

Recently, the CAP has introduced an online service for extracting proficiency testing (PT) results from the same DI middleware mentioned earlier and sending it to the CAP server. This online process will eventually create a system whereby PT specimens flow through the automated testing process (including autoverification) just as QC and patient specimens do. PT data, captured in DI, may be sent directly to a CAP server (similar to QC data sent to the BioRad server) for generation of PT peer comparisons. Hence, PT specimen testing and resulting will be handled as all other specimens as required by CAP. The author's institution has already determined that the most frequent cause of error occurs when results are transcribed off of instrument printouts or CRTs and entered into CAP data input sheets and electronic transmittal screens.

Automating this process will reduce clerical errors as long as all coding and software configuration is correct and tested. As part of the PT result submission process, CAP will require test methods to be LOINC (Logical Object Identifier Naming Code) coded. As part of the broader strategy, laboratories should LOINC code their tests in the LIS because soon it will be required by regulatory and reimbursement agencies.

HARDWARE SUPPORT FOR AUTOVERIFICATION

An increasing array of sophisticated client server computers continues to dominate IT in large enterprise systems. The hardware configuration of these client servers has evolved from *physical* client servers to *virtual* client servers over the last 10 years. Virtual servers are able to serve a large number of software applications across the enterprise rather than have specifically loaded applications running on a designated physical server. Sharing or the virtualization of client servers has increased the capacity on an enterprise basis to keep up with greatly expanding computer cycle needs. Rows of virtual client server hardware dominate computer hardware space in most data centers as exemplified on the Geisinger Health System campus in Danville, Pennsylvania (**Figs. 5** and **6**).

The installation and maintenance of client server hardware is in the domain of IT specialists within most health care organizations. Laboratorians must understand that specific brands, hardware types, operating systems, licensing requirements, and many other factors go in to this maintenance and support. Health information departments are highly conscious of the hardware support issues and have their own strategic plans for rolling out client server hardware. A key component in this plan is maintaining cyber security behind a safe firewall. The enterprise IT department is also responsible for disaster recovery and backup systems in the virtual and physical data center. A separate off-campus lights-out facility with separate servers

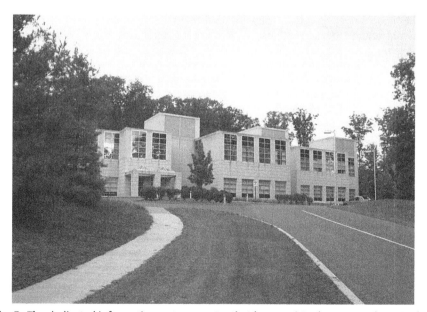

Fig. 5. The dedicated information systems center that houses virtual servers and most other network-terminated devices on the Danville campus of the Geisinger Health System in Danville, Pennsylvania.

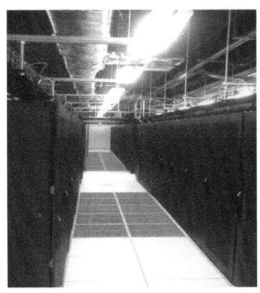

Fig. 6. A portion of the virtual server array in the Geisinger Health System information systems center in Danville, Pennsylvania. This photograph shows one of many rows of servers on a hollow floor with massive air conditioning and fire suppression overhead.

safeguards and backs up the primary server, which, as previously mentioned, is a critical device for maintaining interfaces for all instruments across the enterprise. Applying software and security patches is a monthly chore that IT departments undertake to keep server hardware/software up to date. Laboratorians must respect how important and sophisticated these factors are in overall enterprise informatics. The client server farm is best maintained by an organization's IT professionals with collaboration from the laboratory rather than the laboratory going on its own or insisting that the laboratory's vendor dictate hardware requirements and support.

The network behind the firewall of an enterprise is defined as an intranet (or INFO-web in the Geisinger Health System). The interoperability of multiple client server-based applications exists on this stable robust network. In the Geisinger DI application shown in **Fig. 2**, client servers in the data center apply BioRad, DI, Sunquest, and soon CAP proficiency testing interoperability on a real-time basis.

The laboratory's middleware vendors must understand up front that they must collaborate not just with the laboratory but with the laboratory's IT department as devices are integrated on networks. Middleware vendors must get permission and follow IT protocol to get network access for applying their own particular patches and upgrades. Network access by vendors is defined in policy with well-documented communication logs and contact information. The network must never be unattended while vendors or their subcontractors log onto the network behind the firewall. It has become a routine practice to have bimonthly conference calls with multiple vendors, IT staff, and laboratory staff as upgrades occur to interoperable middleware systems. It is important strategically that the right parties communicate regularly as a group to install and maintain these multiparty interoperable systems. Good project management practices are key to facilitate progress to more sophisticated global autoverification systems.

Imperative in developing a broad enterprise strategic plan for expanding autoverification is understanding how it will evolve in the future and ensuring it will fit into future infrastructure (or info-structure). The aforementioned IICC, working with the IHE, have designed use case scenarios of how this interoperability works from a technical standpoint. Messaging with the use of different actors (eg, instruments, middleware, and LIS) in the use case scenario helps define and give examples of interoperability. It is these use case scenarios, including autoverification, that were demonstrated during the recent (May 2012) IHE/IICC connect-a-thon in Bern, Switzerland. Health care IT professionals understand and appreciate these robust standards, which incorporate messaging specifications broadly used by most enterprise health information systems. Of course, an increased level of understanding IT and information systems is a growing need for laboratorians. Laboratorians as application domain experts must take seriously the responsibility of driving projects for autoverification enhancement and expansion. Understanding application level concepts by perusing the IICC and IHE Web sites and speaking a degree of computer jargon will increase the credibility of laboratorians as they collaborate with their IT counterparts on laboratory connectivity projects. The future will be dominated by laboratorians working with IT staff to improve the functionality of their integrated information systems and especially information systems that provide support for autoverification.

AUTOVERIFICATION PARAMETERS

There are several factors that are programmed in the laboratory information system and/or middleware that except test results from verifying to the LIS.[1,18,23] Terminology is important to define in this process. First of all, the basic process of autoverification is to create rules to *block* or *except* result filing to the LIS. The opposite of *except* is *accept*. The term *autoverification* connotes an *acceptance* process. So even though the basic construct is one of an *except* process, autoverification is discussed as an *accept* process.

Autoverification is the most appropriate term to describe this acceptance process, although the terms *autofiling*, *autovalidation*, and *autocompleting* have also been used. The various parameters used to *except* test results from autoverification include a QC rule failure, high and/or low *verify* limits exceeded, specimen indices exceeded, a shift of patient moving averages, or any other middleware or LIS rule embedded in the instrument to the LIS interface. There is no one correct design but rather traditional and evolving informatics tools to improve the autoverification process. Parameters embedded in the autoverification must filter out poor quality and insure appropriate quality. The key term is *verification* of not just the numerical test result passing an interface but also its parametrically defined correctness. *Autoverification* suggests that the method itself is parametrically defined, the specimen quality is parametrically defined, and the testing process itself is parametrically defined, hence, the test results are as correct as can be expected with these parametric criteria. *Autofiling* suggests that test results are simply filed without parametrically defined quality. *Autocomplete* is another loose term that suggests that the testing process is merely complete without qualification rules. *Autovalidation* is another term that falls short of complete correctness. *Validation* is a term typically applied to correctness of the test method itself but does not properly describe the testing process on an individual specimen.

DELTA CHECKS

One of the first autoverification parameters to be used for several decades is the so-called delta check. Delta checks were originally created more to manually verify patient specimen identification rather than as an autoverification parameter. Delta checks used mainly to assure patient specimen identity are more discriminating at the 20% to 50% shift range, both increasing or decreasing from a previous result. Although delta checks are a form of patient specimen QC, a failed rule would be triggered only by a large shift of a patient value from the patient's previous value for a given period. Delta checks, therefore, have limited usefulness for analytical autoverification and, as originally intended, are best to detect a patient misidentification error rather than a very large change or shift in the testing process. There has been little attention paid to delta check values in the last several years because more emphasis has been placed on patient moving averages as an autoverification parameter to quickly detect shifts in the testing process.[24] Delta checking for individual patient misidentification error is useful and is more fully discussed elsewhere in this issue by Straseski and colleagues.

VERIFY LIMITS

A common parameter in most LIS tables is the *verify limit*. Both high and low verify limit tables are typically created in the LIS to set flags by tests that describe the analytical measurement ranges (AMR) of a particular method. These AMR ranges are quite broad and not useful in autoverification. Rather, a separate set of limits used for autoverification may be more arbitrarily assigned in the LIS or middleware. Some laboratories may set limits as narrow as reference ranges; however, these narrow limits are somewhat overstringent in that results in high-volume acute care hospitals frequently generate correct results slightly outside of the reference range. More broad limits may be set based on a CLIA allowable error that are broader than reference ranges but not as broad as critical limits or AMR. For example, reference ranges for serum sodium are 135 to 146 mEq/L and critical limits are 120 to 155 mEq/L. The CLIA total allowable error is 4 mEq/L, which if applied to the reference range would create autoverification limits of 131 to 150 mEq/L. A rationale for this assignment would be that a shift of 4 mEq/L would prevent autoverification of a low value at 131 mEq/L. Intensive care patients with low sodium values between 135 and 132 would continue to autoverify. Laboratories should apply this type of rationale, test by test, to set fixed autoverification limits within the structure of current LIS and middleware information systems. Part of the judgment for setting a given set of fixed autoverification limits should include the clinical sensitivity of a given test applied to the patient population being tested, the stability of the analytical system (ie, how frequently and to what degree does the instrument shift out of QC ranges), and what are operators observing in the automated workflow vis-á-vis a need to revert to manual verification and a pattern of significant bias. A key question to ask when judging the proper autoverification limit to assign to a given test is how could an autoverified test potentially affect patient treatment? Clinical judgment must be applied and frequently reviewed in assigning these limits as standards of practice, reliability of technology, and other autoverification process strategies improve.

In actual practice, verify limits are especially useful on the lower end because formation of fibrin clots and short sampling may erroneously produce a lower result. These artifactually decreased results may be associated with a single or a few specimens and are specimen related as opposed to reagent or calibration related. Verify limits are typically set based on experience and practice, and it is wise to gain input from operators who know their analytical workstation/workflow and can advise on how changing a limit may affect the detection of these specimen errors. A systematic review or survey of established autoverification limits has not been reported.

SERUM INDICES

Another qualification parameter for autoverification is the serum index. Most chemistry analyzers will measure the absorbance of a specimen to determine the presence of lipid (L, lipemia), hemolysis (H, hemoglobin release), or icterus (I, bilirubin). Limits of these absorbances are established by vendors for judging if L, H, or I make the specimen unsuitable for the analysis of a given test. Different vendors use different means to flag serum indices on their instrument. Some report a numerical result and some report symbols or alpha flags. In turn, these instrument flags are handled in various ways by the interface from the instrument. The actual absorbance value may be captured in middleware or the LIS, or the absorbance value may be converted to an instrument flag in middleware or the LIS. Absorbances and/or instrument flags, in turn, are used in autoverification rules to block reporting of the test and assigning a comment that is reported in its place. It is important to know quantitative and informatics aspects of serum indices while designing autoverification rules using them.

More advanced instruments measure and report actual absorbance values of serum indices. These absorbance values may be quite valuable in analyzing L, H, and I interference for several common laboratory tests. The study of this preanalytical specimen quality has only begun, and this measurement tool shows great promise in screening out unsuitable specimens, finding the cause of unsuitable specimen procurement, and improving specimen quality.

In the Geisinger system, absorbance values are collected in the middleware archive and recently have been extracted for analysis and histogrammed (see **Fig. 3**). Ongoing data-mining studies will link histograms of specific serum indices for a specific test to collection location and individual phlebotomist to survey for suboptimal preanalytical specimen quality. Envisioned studies will link the degree of H (ie, H absorbance) to distributions of potassium (K) values. Using large numbers of K results, the author hopes to establish a quantitative relationship between increasing the H index and the K result. By capturing the appropriate form of parametric data and using it in large numbers, the author hopes to find increasing usefulness in creating an evidence basis for autoverification rules rather than just trusting L, H, and I cutoffs listed in vendor package inserts. Laboratorians should constantly strive to validate the basis of their autoverification process rather than using an all-too-convenient canned approach.

There is an ongoing need to improve the preanalytical quality of results that laboratories report. A very common error is the reporting of elevated K caused by red cell leakage. Most laboratorians can cite an incidence of a provider complaint of receiving a critical limit notification of an elevated K, sending a patient to a local emergency room, only to find that the K was normal. The clinical response to this laboratory error creates undue inconvenience and anxiety to both the patient and provider. In most cases, this error can be tracked to not detecting H in the specimen or, even more frequently, cold storage before centrifugation without apparent hemolysis. This pseudohyperkalemia is often created by improperly storing unspun specimens in the refrigerator or ice during transport. A challenge in the future will be to develop autoverification parameters for specimens with suspect preanalytical quality.

Standard LIS comments should replace test results in this autoverification process. Using an enterprise approach with common LIS and middleware systems facilitates standardization. Although there are exceptions to one size fits all in shared comments and other autoverification parameters in the LIS, standardization is much easier to achieve. The collective approach of doing it right once in a shared system is a very valuable tool for establishing best practice.

MIDDLEWARE BOOLEAN RULES

Current middleware with embedded Boolean logic provides a tool for generating many *if: X and/or: Y then: Z* rules for autoverification. Many laboratories have written hundreds of Boolean rules in middleware to help optimize autoverification in their laboratories. It must be pointed out, as mentioned previously, that writing hundreds of autoverification rules also creates the burden of maintaining and testing these rules in a more laboratory-centric informatics support system. Although laboratory-generated middleware rules are extremely helpful, they tend to be unique for each laboratory; common sets of middleware rules are not broadly scripted.

It is likely that even with this trade-off of greater autoverification rule flexibility necessitating more burdensome support, middleware Boolean rules will be more heavily used in the future. As previously discussed, the interoperability of diverse information systems will come into play in the future, which will enable even more complex and useful rules. Current middleware systems operate with information fields available from LIS order upload and instrument output. These fields are limited because most LIS order fields contain only information necessary to specify the patient, time, and test to be done. Other LIS fields, such as patient location, age/gender demographics, requesting physician/location, laboratory collector identification, and so forth, do not pass the instrument orders interface. If these fields are required for Boolean rule operation in middleware, they must be added to the orders interface. Alternatively, middleware can share information with other accessory information systems to form a decision support rule for autoverification or automatic reflexive testing. It is likely that such multiplexed middleware decision support systems will emerge in the future as relational databases relate to one another. It is also likely that middleware archived data will be extracted in real time to create dashboards for a variety of purposes. It is imperative that the foundation for these advanced systems be built with a priori strategy to minimize the complexity and maximize functionality.

It is the Geisinger experience of the past 10 years that providers embrace decision support, especially real-time decision support, to make their practices more efficient. There is little resentment that computers are taking over as long as the provider community vets and approves of the style and substance of the decision support offered. They are supportive of the laboratory autoverifying and automatic ordering of tests to save them time. An example is the Center for Medicare Services' designated lipoprotein panel (total cholesterol, high-density lipoprotein [HDL] cholesterol, triglycerides, calculated low-density lipoprotein [LDL] cholesterol), which have been enhanced to reflexively automatically order direct LDL cholesterol when triglycerides are greater than 400 mg/dL. There is no need for the provider to call in an add-on direct LDL or call patients back for an additional test because an LDL cholesterol is reported as needed. The automatic ordering of direct LDL has improved the overall provider compliance with monitoring risk groups of patients with diabetes and cardiovascular disease. Laboratory efficiency benefits because the reflexive testing is done on the instrument from the same rerouted tube without operator intervention.

MOVING AVERAGES

Embedding algorithms for capturing moving averages of individual tests in middleware has been released in the last few years. Patient moving averages can be quite useful for determining if a calibration shift has occurred within an analytical system.[23] Sophisticated rules for generating patient averages and judging changes in the testing process has involved several different mathematical models and tends to be nonstan-dardized. As more laboratories adopt patient moving averages in their autoverification scheme, the common practice will likely be published. In the meantime, the use of patient moving averages is as much of an art of the practitioner as it is science. It must be mentioned that hematology instruments have used patient moving averages as a central theme in their QC systems for several years, although the practice has only recently been adopted in chemistry laboratories.

A final parameter to be embedded into the autoverification algorithm is QC. QC has been practiced statistically for several generations of laboratorians, but only recently has it served as one of the main parameters for autoverifying patient results. In the current environment of computer automation, one must not think of automated QC producing automatic quality, An ongoing recognition of the predictive power of QC statistics is important in strategically creating a robust autoverification system. The next section discusses this statistical approach to QC as practiced with automated QC packages in detail.

AUTOMATED QC AND AUTOVERIFICATION

As already described, the Geisinger Health System laboratory has taken an automated approach to enterprise QC on a WAN. The enterprise pathway for archiving QC data provides tool sets at multiple locations. The traditional LIS has been supplemented with secondary middleware QC systems that are more instrument system centric. Chemistry, hematology, and blood gas/whole blood instruments all have graphically rich and user-friendly QC systems at the workstation level. These workstation-level QC systems are increasingly supported by a WAN-based client server in a data center. Fundamental to QC archiving, however, is a designated single source of truth for QC data existing as part of the laboratory scientific record. Additionally, LIS archives are maintained very conservatively, with backup and discoverability as the legal labora-tory record.

QC data must match this source of truth as it passes through the various levels of data archiving and storage; however, the legal record is typically found in the LIS. Because the LIS is shared across all laboratory departments, it is important that rotating technologists know how to access QC information at this source-of-truth data level as well as the more immediately available workstation level. For autoverifi-cation rule assignment and triggering, the LIS controls excepting patient chemistry test results on QC failure in the Geisinger system.

QC FREQUENCY

QC policy needs to describe not just what QC materials are used for what tests but also their frequency of use. The frequency of running QC is most largely determined by the stability of the analytical system, (ie, instrument and reagent) and, as such, needs to be made part of the operating procedure. The frequency of running QC is usually established around look-back requirements of patient results should QC failure occur. Look back on QC failure typically goes back to previous successful QC results. With increasing volumes of chemistry tests performed on high-throughput instruments, the frequency of QC is typically 2 to 4 hours during a 24-hour continuous operation. Description of minimum acceptable QC run frequency of once per shift or once per day typically will not meet the quality needs of a high-volume laboratory. Policy for QC should be set up around practical consid-erations based at least partly on operator experience. QC should not be set up to meet only minimal requirements for accreditation.

QC SYSTEM COORDINATION

QC should also be strategically organized across the system such that laboratory-to-laboratory comparison can be performed. System-wide coordination of using single lot numbers; creating consistent site-neutral QC policy; and, most importantly, reviewing the data for a system quality standard require set-aside resources and time. System-wide QC basis is not simply standardizing bench tasks by operators running instruments; QC needs to be reviewed to validate that quality is in control and site neutral across the system. Several of the aforementioned information system tools are used and will be increasingly used for this system coordination. The results from enterprise QC in the Geisinger system are viewable not only in monthly peer comparisons but also in real time for operators and supervisors from each laboratory. System coordination also involves looking for means to improve, and it is important for groups of stakeholders to meet and discuss what the next enhancement might be. In the Geisinger system, the Advanced Analytical QC Committee serves this role.

SPECIMEN MICROCLOTS

Practices for judging that testing is in control need to be established along with the aforementioned autoverification parameters. QC of the analytical system (eg, instrument and reagent) should not be the sole means for autoverifying a patient result. QC may judge the acceptability of testing by statistically measuring the analytical system but does not detect problems associated with a single patient specimen (eg, microclots) or a series of patient specimens. Unlike serum index, which is measureable, partial occlusion of a specimen probe causing a decreased test result often goes undetected. It is reasonable to expect that in the future instrument flags or error messages detecting increased specimen probe pressure may be passed to associated middleware for autoverification rule triggering. Problems that they are, microclots can affect adjoining tests and specimens. Autoverification parameters need to be established to judge the acceptability of a specimen when a panel of tests are run from a single tube; if only one of the panel tests fails autoverification, other tests from the specimen also need to be excepted (ie, specimen-specific autoverification).

DASHBOARDS

Because the amount of real-time data presented to operators of high-volume laboratory instruments can be overwhelming, graphic human-friendly displays need to be considered. The raw data residing in middleware may be reduced to create visual dashboards that aid in establishing and monitoring QC autoverification rules. An example is shown in **Fig. 4** for ongoing monitoring of sigmas for a single test (eg, K) that has a relatively high sigma. One can see patterns and trends much more clearly in a single glance as opposed to analyzing columns and rows of numerical data. The consistently high sigmas shown for all practice sites using harmonized K ion selective electrodes show a safe margin for establishing 1-3S rules as opposed to 1-2S rules.

FUNCTIONAL AUTOVERIFICATION

This dashboard approach is a form of data reduction that makes an overall affiliated system more comprehendible than reams of affiliate QC reports. By dashboard monitoring sigmas of general chemistry tests, the Geisinger system has created far fewer false QC run rejections and not suffered reduced quality as graded by CAP proficiency testing. **Table 1** shows that 76.9% fewer QC run rejections occurred after a sigma approach was taken to QC rules establishment in general chemistry workstation

GML Tests Qc'ed	Before Sigma QC Rejects	Total QC Points	Before Sigma QC Reject (%)	After Sigma QC Rejects	Total QC Points	After Sigma QC Reject (%)
ALKP	108	2372	4.55	2	2599	0.08
K	47	4589	1.02	17	3058	0.56
AMY	31	1107	2.80	11	1613	0.68
HDL	25	1358	1.84	10	1211	0.83
LDL	36	482	7.47	4	543	0.74
CK	80	1332	6.01	38	1741	2.18
LIPA	17	950	1.79	6	1341	0.45
AST	73	2588	2.82	17	2821	0.60
TBILI	36	1468	2.45	2	1399	0.14
LD	2	409	0.49	2	714	0.28
TRIG	120	1411	8.50	3	1202	0.25
URIC	2	409	0.49	0	654	0.00
GLU	70	706	9.92	5	694	0.72
TOTAL	455	16655	2.73	105	14927	0.70
Reduction (%)				76.92		

Table 1
Use of sigma analysis to reduce general chemistry QC rejections before and after changing of QC rules (1-2s rules to 1-3s rules)

Abbreviations: AKLP, alkaline phosphatase; AMY, amylase; AST, aspartate transaminase; CK, creatinine kinase; GLU, glucose; GML, Geisinger Medical Laboratory; LD, lactate dehydrogenase; LIPA, lipase; QC'ed, quality controlled; TBILI, total bilirubin; TRIG, triglyceride; URIC, uric acid.

autoverification. This dramatic reduction was observed in all WAN-connected chemistry instruments at all testing sites in the affiliated enterprise.

Similar approaches for less stringent QC rules leading to fewer false run rejections have been demonstrated with more clinical approaches to QC.[24] Whether by the use of sigma analysis or more broad QC ranges based on clinical impact, fewer false run rejections have a very positive effect on workflow in the laboratory. A false QC run rejection leads to the discontinuation of autoverification until the out-of-control condition is corrected. During this time, numerous patient specimens are not candidates for autoverification; manual or halted results verification leads to a delay in result reporting.

The disruption to autoverification by false QC run rejection or other autoverification parameters has not been reported. If autoverification by specimen (not just tests) is followed, one may have a relatively high *apparent* autoverification rate (eg, 70%–90%); however, the actual time spent autoverifying may be considerably less. The time percentage in autoverification mode at the workstation is a better measurement of functional autoverification than merely accounting the percentage of tests that are candidates for autoverification.

SUMMARY

Although still largely practiced as an efficiency tool at the laboratory instrument workstation level, autoverification is rapidly expanding with increased functionality provided by middleware tools. It is imperative that autoverification of laboratory test results be viewed as a process evolving into a much broader, more sophisticated form of decision support, which will require strategic planning to form a foundational tool set for the laboratory. The introduction and integration of middleware by several instrument vendors has already accelerated widespread implementation of more sophisticated autoverification. One must strategically plan to expand autoverification in the more distant future to include a vision of IGO interfaces, reflexive testing, and interoperability with other information systems. It is hoped that the observations, examples, and opinions expressed in this article will stimulate such short-term and long-term strategic planning.

REFERENCES

1. Duca DJ. Autoverification in a laboratory information system. Lab Med 2002; 33(1):21–5.
2. Jones JB. The electronic health record: improving best practice. Bulletin Royal Col Pathology 2007;137:38–41.
3. Felder R. Laboratory reporting for the future: linking autoverification to the electronic medical record. American Association for Clinical Chemistry. AACC Continuing Education. Available at: http://www.aacc.org/resourcecenters/archivedprograms/expert_access/2004/record/Pages/default.aspx#.
4. CLSI C24A3. Statistical quality control for quantitative measurement procedures. Wayne (PA): Clinical and Laboratory Standards Institute; 2006.
5. The Joint Commission. Failure modes and effects analysis in health care: proactive risk reduction. Oakbrook Terrace (IL): The Joint Commission, Oakbrook Terrace; 2010.
6. CLSI EP23A. Laboratory quality control based on risk management. Wayne (PA): Clinical and Laboratory Standards Institute; 2011.
7. CMS memorandum: implementing the Individualized Quality Control Plan (IQCP) for Clinical Laboratory Improvement Amendments (CLIA). March 9, 2012.
8. ISO 15189. Medical laboratories – particular requirements for quality and competence. Geneva (Switzerland): ISO; 2007.
9. CLSI EP18A2. Risk management techniques to identify and control laboratory error sources. 2nd edition. Wayne (PA): Clinical and Laboratory Standards Institute; 2009.
10. CMS memorandum: initial plans and policy implementation for Clinical and Laboratory Standards Institute (CLSI) Evaluation Protocol-23 (EP), "Laboratory quality control based on risk management," as Clinical Laboratory Improvement Amendment (CLIA) quality control (QC) policy. November 4, 2011.
11. Shih M-C, Chang H-M, Tien N, et al. Building and validating an autoverification system in the clinical chemistry laboratory. Lab Med 2011;42:668–73, v.
12. Rao LV, Okorodudu AO. Integrated automation in the clinical chemistry. In: Lewandrowski K, editor. Clinical chemistry: laboratory management and clinical correlations. New York: Lippincott; 2002. p. 205–11.
13. Pearlman ES, Bilello L, Stauffer J, et al. Implications of autoverification for the clinical laboratory. Clin Leadersh Manag Rev 2002;16:237–9.
14. Hoffman J, Jones JB, Olson E, Improving instrument communication: the IICC will help all laboratory instruments, technology speak the same language. Advance for administrators of the laboratory. Available at: http://laboratory-manager.advanceweb.com/Features/Articles/Better-Communication-Between-Lab-Instruments.aspx. Accessed October 13, 2010.
15. American Society for Testing and Materials. Standard specification for transferring information between clinical instruments and computer systems. Conshohocken, PA: ASTM 1394-91.

16. CLSI Standards Organization. Autoverification of clinical laboratory test resulting approved guideline (Auto 10-A). Wayne (PA): Clinical Laboratory Standards Institute; 2006.
17. Jones JB, Yost J, Parl F. Webinar, improving the electronic exchange of lab information, (CD ROM). Washington, DC: American Association for Clinical Chemistry; 2010.
18. Torke N, Borai L, Nguyen T, et al. Process improvement and operational efficiency through test results autoverification. Clin Chem 2005;51:2406–8.
19. Jones JB, Sargent D, Young D, et al. Integration of a multisite enterprise quality control program on a wide area network and use of sigma statistics to standardize Westgard rules. Clin Chem 2011;57:8 A117.
20. Westgard JO. Six sigma risk analysis: designing analytic QC plans for the medical laboratory. Madison (WI): Westgard QC, Inc.; 2011.
21. Jones JB, Sargent D, Young D, et al. Use of networked Westgard advisor quality control software to reduce false QC rejections in a regional laboratory system. Clin Chem 2012;58:10 A56.
22. Westgard JO. Charts of operational process specifications ("OPSpecs charts") for assessing the precision, accuracy, and quality control needed to satisfy proficiency testing performance criteria. Clin Chem 1992;38:1226–33.
23. Johnson J, Stelmach D. Autoverification of test results. Clinical Laboratory News 2007;33(9).
24. Westgard JO, Smith FA, Mountain PJ, et al. Design and assessment of average of normal (AON) patient data algorithms to maximize run lengths for automatic process control. Clin Chem 1996;42:1683–8.

Patient Safety & Post-analytical Error

Stacy E. Walz, PhD, MT(ASCP)[a], Teresa P. Darcy, MD, MMM[b],*

KEYWORDS

- Post-analytical • Post-post-analytical • Test result management
- Electronic health record

KEY POINTS

- Laboratories must continue to assess the post-analytical phase of the total testing process using monitors, such as critical call notification, turnaround time, changed reports, and accuracy of result transmission from the laboratory information system across interfaces and in paper reports.
- Laboratories must become advocates for patient safety by developing new quality monitors to ensure that results posting in electronic health records are interpretable and are received and reviewed by responsible providers of care.
- The explosion of environments in which laboratory results are displayed, such as smart phones, tablets, and patient portals, make the management of test results an increasingly error-prone process.
- High-risk transitions of care, such as patients being discharged from the hospital with pending laboratory tests, should be a focus for developing new quality processes and monitors.

POST-ANALYTICAL ERROR

Traditionally, the laboratory community has viewed post-analytical errors as errors that occur after the analysis is complete but within the confines of the 4 walls of the laboratory itself and under the control of the laboratory. Activities that fall into the post-analytical phase of the total testing process (TTP) include result reporting, critical value notification, manual transcription of results and subsequent data entry, and analysis of turnaround times (TAT).[1–4]

The post-analytic phase of the TTP has been thought to be less prone to error than the preanalytical phase because of the widespread adoption of technology and automated results reporting. In a summary of available data on error rates in the laboratory,

Disclosure statement: The authors have no relevant financial relationships to disclose.
[a] Department of Clinical Laboratory Sciences, Arkansas State University, PO Box 910, State University, AR 72467, USA; [b] Department of Pathology and Laboratory Medicine, University of Wisconsin School of Medicine and Public Health, 600 Highland Avenue, B4/251, Madison, WI 53792-2472, USA
* Corresponding author.
E-mail address: tdarcy@uwhealth.org

Clin Lab Med 33 (2013) 183–194
http://dx.doi.org/10.1016/j.cll.2012.10.001
0272-2712/13/$ – see front matter © 2013 Elsevier Inc. All rights reserved.

labmed.theclinics.com

Nevalainen and colleagues[5] found an error rate of 0.0477% in the reporting of test results or 477 defects per million results. This finding is a sigma metric of 4.80, which is considered an excellent process in health care and far better than most preanalytical processes.

POST-POST-ANALYTICAL ERROR

In this new era of health care with the widespread adoption of electronic health records and the focus on the continuum of patient care and quality outcomes, laboratory professionals are being asked to think outside the 4 walls of the laboratory and consider errors that involve the interface between the laboratory result and the clinician. A new term coined for this part of the resulting process is post-post-analytical.[6] The post-post-analytical process can be thought of as closing the brain-to-brain loop,[1,7] which begins when the clinician initially thinks about which test to order and ends when the test result has been received, interpreted, and acted on. In 2011, the National Quality Forum added 2 new laboratory-related errors to its list of serious reportable events.[8] These events are patient death or serious injury resulting from the irretrievable loss of an irreplaceable biologic specimen and patient death or serious injury resulting from the failure to follow up or communicate laboratory, pathology, or radiology test results.[9]

These post-post-analytical errors[6] were once thought of as beyond the direct control of the laboratory and in the realm of the clinician. Risk management demands that laboratories take an active role in understanding and managing patient safety risks beyond traditional post-analytical errors and into the post-post-analytical phase of the total testing process.

Patient safety initiatives have been popping up left and right after the Institute of Medicine (IOM) highlighted rather frightening data on medical errors in their publication *To Err is Human*.[10] Another IOM publication, *Crossing the Quality Chasm*,[11] went on to describe 6 aims for quality patient care, including timeliness, safety, patient centeredness, efficiency, effectiveness, and equitability. Most researchers recognize that improving the quality of patient care will require interdisciplinary conversation and a variety of problem-solving tactics. There is no magic bullet that will solve this problem single handedly.

This article discusses traditional post-analytical quality controls and hazard identification in the management of laboratory test results. Additional topics in this article are the display and interpretation of results; the routing of results; and high-risk transitions of patient care, including pending test results at the time of hospital discharge.[12–14]

REQUIREMENTS FOR MONITORING THE POST-ANALYTICAL PROCESS

The Clinical Laboratory Improvement Amendments (CLIA) dictate that laboratories must monitor and evaluate the overall quality of post-analytic systems and correct identified problems.[15] The standards in the "Post-analytical Systems" section are brief. The laboratory must assure that results are accurately and reliably sent to the final report destination. The standards address the content of the test result report, referred testing, as well as the changed result and critical result. Laboratories must have ongoing mechanisms to monitor; assess; and, when indicated, correct problems identified in the post-analytical phase of the TTP.

Recommendations for quality monitors for post-analytical systems are included in the standards for laboratory accreditation.[7] Because monitoring relates to the post-analytical phase, standard 2 of the International Patient Safety Goals of The Joint Commission (TJC) requires the laboratory to develop an approach to improve the communication among caregivers, particularly regarding critical result reporting protocols. The College of American Pathologists (CAP) Laboratory Accreditation Program's checklist requires monitoring of quality indicators, such as critical value reporting and short turn-around time (STAT) test TAT, as well as processes, such as accuracy of data transmission across electronic interfaces. Like TJC, the CAP stipulates 4 laboratory patient safety goals, all of which involve activities outside the analytical phase of testing. Although the International Standards Organization (ISO) is less prescriptive than the other accrediting bodies, it does describe monitoring and management activities related to post-analytical errors.[16]

DETECTION AND MEASUREMENT OF POST-ANALYTICAL ERRORS

It is difficult to measure the prevalence of post-analytical errors of any type, which also makes it difficult to directly link laboratory errors and patient safety. The TTP is complex and involves a variety of different professions and settings.[1] With so many variables, it becomes hard to pinpoint a single reason or explanation for why a medical error was made. There is no standardized definition or denominators for laboratory errors,[17,18] which makes comparison among studies virtually impossible. Particularly for the post-analytical errors that occur outside the 4 walls of the laboratory, there is inconsistent interpretation of the roles and responsibilities in monitoring those errors; good, standardized measures are not readily available.[19,20]

As more and more anecdotal and research evidence surfaces regarding post-analytical errors and patient safety in general, several groups have been working diligently to address the problem. The International Federation of Clinical Chemistry and Laboratory Medicine has an active working group on laboratory errors and patient safety[7,21] that is creating a systematic common reporting system based on standardized data collection. Post-analytical quality specifications include the percentage of laboratory reports delivered outside the specified time frame, the percentage of critical values successfully communicated, and the average amount of time it takes to communicate those critical values.

The Centers for Disease Control and Prevention held the Institute on Critical Issues in Health Laboratory Practice in 2007[22] to discuss how to advance collaborative care among the laboratory, providers, and payers by enhancing communication, defining and measuring quality parameters that link laboratory service performance with patient outcomes, and preparing for future expectations and contributions of the laboratory to patient care. Four major recommendations came out of this institute:

- Further scholarly work should focus on preanalytic and post-analytic phases of the TTP.
- Nonlaboratory stakeholders in improvement need to be identified.
- Partnerships with health information technology experts and laboratory information system (LIS) manufacturers should be made to solve information technology (IT) barriers and problems.
- Laboratory professionals at all levels need to be educated about health services research, quality improvement, and patient safety.

THE POST-ANALYTICAL PROCESS

One of the most important challenges for laboratory professionals will be to assist in the management of patient test results. This assistance requires an expansion of the role of the laboratory. It is no longer enough to send our test results across an interface to an electronic record or call a critical result and assume our work is done. There is an often-quoted statistic that 70% of medical decisions are based on diagnostic test results, including laboratory or imaging.[23] The breakdown in the handoff of information in the care of patients is a common underlying cause of medical error. In TJC database on sentinel events, breakdown in communication among caregivers is the most commonly identified root cause in sentinel events associated with a delay in treatment and is among the top 3 root causes for all sentinel event types.[24] Failure to follow up test results is cited as one of the more common causes of medical malpractice lawsuits.[25-28]

Fig. 1 shows the map for the post-analytical process that must occur to ensure that patients receive an appropriate follow-up of test results. The first step in this process is the accurate and timely communication of the test result by the laboratory. This step is under the direct and sole control of the laboratory. That results are received by the appropriate or correct provider and interpreted correctly are process steps that require laboratory and clinical processes to be integrated. That test results are reviewed and appropriate follow-up completed can be considered clinical processes into which the laboratory has little input. Patient safety requires all steps in the new post-analytical process to be completed.

Post-analytical process
- Communication of result by laboratory
- Result received by correct provider
- Result reviewed
- Result interpreted correctly
- Result follow-up appropriate to patient

COMMUNICATION OF TEST RESULTS

The first type of post-analytical process failure is that the laboratory does not properly communicate the result. This issue might be an accuracy or timeliness issue.

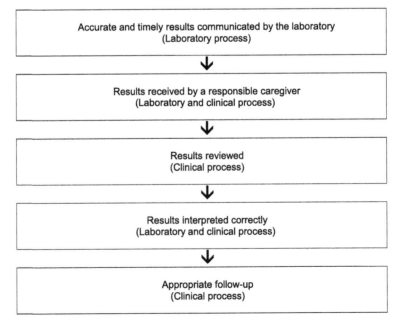

Fig. 1. Post-analytical process.

Laboratories should review indicators and existing quality monitors to address these potential failures. Failures in this step include the following:

Failures in communication of test results
- Tests performed but not reported
- Patient identification error in results reporting
- Delay in reporting
- Incorrect calculation
- Critical result notification failed or delayed
- Results not sent because of communication failures

Instruments and the LIS provide tools for the laboratory to monitor that tests performed are resulted or reported through the use of review lists and pending test monitors. Identification errors that occur in the results reporting step are most often found in areas of the laboratory that are less automated and have manual reporting. Requiring a 2-step process for any manual test result, auditing results that are entered manually into the LIS, and monitoring corrected results or variance reports are several methods of identifying results that have been reported on the wrong patient because of an identification error at the resulting step.[29]

Laboratories monitor TAT for testing. TAT may be monitored from the point of specimen collection to result reporting or from the receipt of the specimen in the laboratory to result reporting. TAT monitors may be selected for high-volume tests, low-volume tests, or for those tests for which the laboratory has had complaints. A variety of TAT monitors for key clinical services or tests should be selected. TAT goals should be established; if the goal is not being met, action plans should be developed. Benchmarking data for TAT are available for several tests and service areas.[30,31]

The timeliness of the critical result notification is a standard post-analytical process quality control, and benchmarking data are available for this process. This monitoring often includes timeliness and completeness of the call and may include the critical call abandonment rate, that is, the failure to reach a responsible caregiver as outlined in the laboratory or hospital policy.[32]

Table 1 describes potential failures in the communication of test results and common quality monitors used by laboratories today.

TEST RESULTS COMMUNICATED BUT NOT RECEIVED

In the first article of its kind, Yackel and Embi[33] examined unintended errors in the management of test results in the electronic health record, focusing on the reasons

Table 1
Potential failures in the communication of test results and laboratory monitors

Failure	Monitor
Tests performed but not reported	Review lists
Patient identification error in results reporting	Corrected reports/variance
Delay in reporting	TAT monitor
Incorrect calculation	Verification of calculations
Critical result notification failed or delayed	Critical call timeliness
Results not sent because of communication failures	Interface error monitor

why results communicated from the laboratory were never received. They identified 4 distinct categories of errors resulting in a test result sent but not received by the correct caregiver.

Failure modes in electronic receipt of results
- Logic errors in interface and results routing
- Provider record issues
- Electronic health record (EHR) system settings
- System maintenance–related errors

Results routing in the electronic health record is a complex proposition and sometimes implemented without sufficient knowledge of laboratory processes or without the input of the laboratory. Yackel and Embi[33] report that the design of routing suppressed all inpatient results from the provider inbox, but the anatomic pathology LIS did not distinguish inpatient from ambulatory. As a result, by default, all anatomic pathology results were considered inpatient and, thus, suppressed from inbox routing to ambulatory providers. Similarly, a clinic might ask for routing logic for microbiology results, but what is considered a microbiology result to a clinician is not how those tests are classified in the LIS.

A surprising number of provider record issues were identified that caused a failure in the receipt of results. These issues included the mismatching of LIS and EHR provider tables and the failure to inactivate an inbox account for departed providers. Recommendations for improved systems included developing error queues when results cannot be delivered electronically and tracking mechanisms for critical tests, such as cancer diagnostics. As errors occur and are analyzed, the laboratory can participate in specific testing and validation of result receipt after, for example, system changes or upgrades.

RESULTS NOT REVIEWED

Laboratories are not directly responsible for ensuring that all reported test results have been reviewed. In May of 2011, a kidney transplant program in the United States was voluntarily shut down following a failure to follow up on a laboratory test result. The results of a positive hepatitis C test sat in a living kidney donor's medical record for more than 2 months before her kidney was transplanted into a man who did not have the virus, according to the findings of a federal investigation into the case.[34] But despite at least 6 chances to review the test result and possibly stop the transplant because of the potentially lethal hepatitis C infecting the donor, none of the doctors or nurses involved in the case did so, according to the Centers for Medicare and Medicaid Services' investigation.

Although not directly responsible, laboratories might participate in the organizational design of systems designed to monitor the reviewing of results within a specified timeframe, involving automatic or manual tracking systems to provide reminders or to escalate the issue. In addition, organizations should develop policies outlining which provider is responsible for the review of results, particularly when electronic systems easily route a single result to multiple providers.

The old adage *no news is good news* does not support patient safety in our current health care environment. Direct notification of patients of their test results as part of the Accountable Care Act adds one more layer of safety in the reporting of laboratory test results. If there is a failure of the provider who has received the test result to review it, the patient has also received the result and can follow up with the provider.

RESULTS NOT INTERPRETED CORRECTLY

Patient safety is getting the right laboratory result to the right person at the right time in a usable/interpretable format. The electronic health record enables large quantities of data to be sent from the laboratory to a variety of environments and displays. The following are just some of the areas of the EHR where laboratory results may be displayed:

- Chart equivalent: report of an individual test or panel
- Cumulative/chronologic view, such as the EHR patient summary record
- Discharge summaries
- Emergency department tracking board
- Flow sheets
- Patient letters
- Patient portals: Web based and smart phone or tablet based
- Data pulled through community exchanges
- Smart phone and tablet applications

Laboratories may have a validated display of results in one or more of these areas but most laboratories do not have the resources to validate all. The laboratory may not have been included in the decision to implement these applications. But if given the opportunity before or after implementation, the laboratory should be prepared with a checklist of test results to quickly see if major problems exist in the display of results. Result displays should be reviewed for presence and accuracy of the following:

- Result/value
- Units of measure
- Reference range
- Collection date/time
- Flags: abnormality, changed, critical
- Laboratory comments
- Performing laboratory site
- Trailing zeros
- Report date

Not all of these elements will be viewable on the same screen in the display being studied in the record, but they should all be retrievable. In addition, laboratories should pay particular attention to viewing some of the following types of results: corrected and multi-corrected results, microbiology organism identification and susceptibility, anatomic pathology, and table-based flow cytometry results. If the organization has multiple laboratory sites performing the same tests, the displays across laboratories should be reviewed. Reference ranges from the performing laboratory are critical in this scenario.

Laboratories should carefully review any physician complaint or patient safety event related to the display of laboratory results. In the experience of one author (Darcy), several areas of concern have been identified. Important attributes of results are sometimes reported as comments. For example, many laboratories report the finding of band neutrophils as a comment to a differential rather than as a discrete component of the differential. For patients with a normal white count, the presence of bands may be overlooked when clinicians are reviewing the discrete laboratory data. Another example is that many electronic records cannot use commas and do not justify columns of data at the decimal point. For large amounts of numeric data, a tumor marker of a result of 2220 may be misinterpreted as 22220 and vice versa.

HIGH-RISK GAPS IN APPROPRIATE FOLLOW-UP OF TEST RESULTS

Failure to follow up on test results is not a new problem and is an underlying factor in many medical malpractice lawsuits. The frequency of the failure to follow up on laboratory test results in an ambulatory setting varies from 2% to 50% among primary care providers.[35]

A very high-risk safety gap for patients occurs at the discharge of patients from the hospital. Two types of errors occur: the failure to review and follow up on results of tests that were pending at the time of the discharge and the failure of patients to receive the diagnostic tests that were ordered for the postdischarge period. Baseline data before implementation of an electronic health record indicate that 35.9% of the recommended postdischarge procedures are not completed.[36]

In a study of laboratory results pending at hospital discharge, one of the authors (Walz) found 32% of patients had test results pending at the time of discharge, yet only 11% of discharge summaries documented the pending tests.[13] Patients most often left the hospital with pending microbiology cultures and reference laboratory tests. Ong and colleagues[37] found that although tests ordered on the day of the patient discharge represented only 7% of all tests ordered during the admission, 21% of these tests were never followed up. Nearly 15% of all tests not followed up in this study had abnormal results, which could contribute to both adverse events and increased risk of readmission.

TOOLS TO ADDRESS POST-ANALYTICAL ERRORS IN THE LABORATORY

Many tools exist to assist laboratories in identifying and correcting post-analytical errors. The Clinical Laboratory Standards Institute's document on risk assessment (EP23A) is the newest tool available, even though it is based on concepts that have been actively and successfully used in manufacturing for decades but are somewhat new concepts to the laboratory. This document instructs laboratories in identifying both human and system factors that can fail in the total testing process, both inside and outside the laboratory's 4 walls, and recommends that laboratories introduce measures that quickly detect and rectify problems. The document helps laboratories widen their focus to consider activities outside their immediate control.

Many of the existing tools used in manufacturing for identifying human and system factors influencing a process can be adapted for the laboratory setting. These tools include process control analysis and proactive hazards analysis, such as failure modes and effects analysis (**Fig. 2**).[38] Techniques more familiar to the laboratory include quality-improvement tools, such as Six Sigma, ISO quality systems, and total quality management.[39]

Once factors with the potential to negatively influence the testing process are identified, strategic planning can ensue to identify steps to address those factors and launch an agenda for change. Particularly in this era when the laboratory is being asked to consider errors that occur outside its direct control, it is paramount for the laboratory to establish a seat at that multidisciplinary table for patient safety discussions.[40–42]

Advances in IT offer many powerful, potential solutions for post-analytical errors.[43–45] IT can readily identify and track problems relating to result reporting, critical value reporting, and TAT. Even for post-post-analytical errors that involve the laboratory-clinician interface, IT can be a powerful tool. The body of evidence is growing and supporting the use of IT in post-analytical situations. The provision of patient-specific, expert-driven interpretation of test results[6,46–48] is one way the laboratory can aid

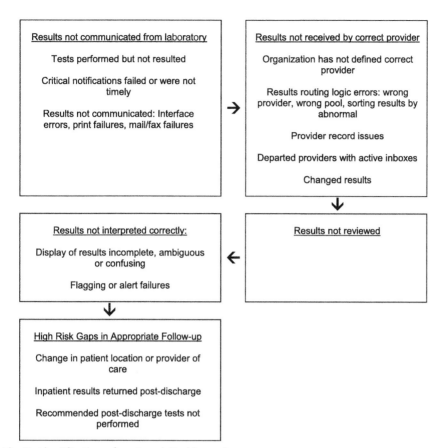

Fig. 2. Identification of post-analytical hazards.

physicians at this interface. Although less technical methods exist (think phone calls or face-to-face conversations), IT, such as e-mail, electronic alerts, and smart phone applications, is widely used to tackle these situations.

SUMMARY

Health care in general is at a pivotal juncture in this country. With mandates for use of information technology, financial penalties imposed on hospitals when patients bounce back into the system within 30 days, and the potential of a national health care system (just to name a few big changes), health care professionals and facilities are scrambling to reduce costs, improve quality, and stay in business.

The laboratory is also at a pivotal point. For years we have made great progress in improving the safety of the post-analytical process through the widespread adoption of automation and result interfaces. With the advent of the electronic health record, laboratory professionals are called to be patient safety advocates beyond the post-analytical and into the post-post-analytical process. Laboratory professionals generate large quantities of data that are critical for patient care. Now our challenge is to turn that data into usable information by ensuring that accurate and interpretable results are sent, received, and interpreted by the clinician responsible for the care of the patients.

Post-post-analytical quality control demands we participate in process design and monitoring for our test results, particularly in those areas known to be high risk for patients, such as hospital discharge. But with the realization that health care's patient safety problems are multifactorial and that no profession is an island and singly capable of solving these problems, now is the time for the laboratory to get involved in the conversations, brainstorming, and solutions to mitigate the risks of harm to our patients.

REFERENCES

1. Plebani M. The detection and prevention of errors in laboratory medicine. Ann Clin Biochem 2010;47(Pt 2):101–10.
2. Plebani M. Errors in clinical laboratories or errors in laboratory medicine? Clin Chem Lab Med 2006;44(6):750–9.
3. Plebani M. Exploring the iceberg of errors in laboratory medicine. Clin Chim Acta 2009;404(1):16–23.
4. Kalra J. Medical errors: impact on clinical laboratories and other critical areas. Clin Biochem 2004;37(12):1052–62.
5. Nevalainen D, Berte L, Kraft C, et al. Evaluating laboratory performance on quality indicators with the six sigma scale. Arch Pathol Lab Med 2000;124(4):516–9.
6. Laposata M, Dighe A. "Pre-pre" and "post-post" analytical error: high-incidence patient safety hazards involving the clinical laboratory. Clin Chem Lab Med 2007;45(6):712–9.
7. Hawkins R. Managing the pre- and post-analytical phases of the total testing process. Ann Lab Med 2012;32(1):5–16.
8. National Quality Forum. Serious reportable events in healthcare 2011 update: a consensus report. Report 2011. Available at: http://www.qualityforum.org/WorkArea/linkit.aspx?LinkIdentifier=id&ItemID=61352.
9. Darcy T. Two new national quality forum serious reportable events focus on clinical labs. How should your laboratory prepare? Clinical Laboratory News 2011;37(10).
10. Kohn LT, Corrigan J, Donaldson MS. To err is human: building a safer health system. Washington, D.C: National Academy Press; 2000. p. xxi, 287.
11. Institute of Medicine (U.S.). Committee on Quality of Health Care in America. Crossing the quality chasm: a new health system for the 21st century. Washington, D.C: National Academy Press; 2001. p. xx, 337.
12. Roy CL, Poon EG, Karson AS, et al. Patient safety concerns arising from test results that return after hospital discharge. Ann Intern Med 2005;143(2):121–8.
13. Walz SE, Smith M, Cox E, et al. Pending laboratory tests and the hospital discharge summary in patients discharged to sub-acute care. J Gen Intern Med 2011;26(4):393–8.
14. Were MC, Li X, Kesterson J, et al. Adequacy of hospital discharge summaries in documenting tests with pending results and outpatient follow-up providers. J Gen Intern Med 2009;24(9):1002–6.
15. Clinical laboratory improvement amendment: Rule number 493.1290, CMS, Legal regulation. 1988. Available at: http://www.cdc.gov/clia/regs/toc.aspx.
16. Shahangian S, Snyder SR. Laboratory medicine quality indicators: a review of the literature. Am J Clin Pathol 2009;131(3):418–31.
17. Plebani M, Sciacovelli L, Lippi G. Quality indicators for laboratory diagnostics: consensus is needed. Ann Clin Biochem 2011;48(Pt 5):479.
18. Plebani M. Towards quality specifications in extra-analytical phases of laboratory activity. Clin Chem Lab Med 2004;42(6):576–7.

19. Montoya ID. Patient safety and quality improvement: a policy assessment. Clin Lab Sci 2010;23(4):212–8.
20. Dintzis SM, Stetsenko GY, Sitlani CM, et al. Communicating pathology and laboratory errors: anatomic pathologists' and laboratory medical directors' attitudes and experiences. Am J Clin Pathol 2011;135(5):760–5.
21. Sciacovelli L, Plebani M. The IFCC Working Group on laboratory errors and patient safety. Clin Chim Acta 2009;404(1):79–85.
22. Grzybicki DM, Shahangian S, Pollock AM, et al. A summary of deliberations on strategic planning for continuous quality improvement in laboratory medicine. Am J Clin Pathol 2009;131(3):315–20.
23. Forsman RW. Why is the laboratory an afterthought for managed care organizations? Clin Chem 1996;42(5):813–6.
24. Database on sentinel events. [cited]; Available at: http://www.jointcommission.org/assets/1/18/Root_Causes_Event_Type_2004_2Q2012.pdf. Accessed October 1, 2012.
25. Casalino LP, Dunham D, Chin MH, et al. Frequency of failure to inform patients of clinically significant outpatient test results. Arch Intern Med 2009;169(12):1123–9.
26. Holohan TV, Colestro J, Grippi J, et al. Analysis of diagnostic error in paid malpractice claims with substandard care in a large healthcare system. South Med J 2005;98(11):1083–7.
27. Singh H, Petersen LA, Thomas EJ. Understanding diagnostic errors in medicine: a lesson from aviation. Qual Saf Health Care 2006;15(3):159–64.
28. Wahls T. Diagnostic errors and abnormal diagnostic tests lost to follow-up: a source of needless waste and delay to treatment. J Ambul Care Manage 2007;30(4):338–43.
29. Nakhleh RE, Zarbo RJ. Amended reports in surgical pathology and implications for diagnostic error detection and avoidance: a College of American Pathologists Q-probes study of 1,667,547 accessioned cases in 359 laboratories. Arch Pathol Lab Med 1998;122(4):303–9.
30. Novis DA, Jones BA, Dale JC, et al. Biochemical markers of myocardial injury test turnaround time: a College of American Pathologists Q-Probes study of 7020 troponin and 4368 creatine kinase-MB determinations in 159 institutions. Arch Pathol Lab Med 2004;128(2):158–64.
31. Steindel SJ. Timeliness of clinical laboratory tests. A discussion based on five College of American Pathologists Q-Probe studies. Arch Pathol Lab Med 1995;119(10):918–23.
32. Howanitz PJ, Steindel SJ, Heard NV. Laboratory critical values policies and procedures: a College of American Pathologists Q-Probes Study in 623 institutions. Arch Pathol Lab Med 2002;126(6):663–9.
33. Yackel TR, Embi PJ. Unintended errors with EHR-based result management: a case series. J Am Med Inform Assoc 2010;17(1):104–7.
34. Hamill SD. Transplant error finds more at fault: a probe into the UPMC kidney transplant error found a nephrologist was also to blame. Pittsburgh (PA): Pittsburgh Post Gazette; 2011.
35. Murff HJ, Gandhi TK, Karson AK, et al. Primary care physician attitudes concerning follow-up of abnormal test results and ambulatory decision support systems. Int J Med Inform 2003;71(2–3):137–49.
36. Moore C, McGinn T, Halm E. Tying up loose ends: discharging patients with unresolved medical issues. Arch Intern Med 2007;167(12):1305–11.
37. Ong MS, Magrabi F, Jones G, et al. Last orders: follow-up of tests ordered on the day of hospital discharge. Arch Intern Med 2012;1–2.

38. Signori C, Ceriotti F, Sanna A, et al. Process and risk analysis to reduce errors in clinical laboratories. Clin Chem Lab Med 2007;45(6):742–8.

39. Plebani M. Errors in laboratory medicine and patient safety: the road ahead. Clin Chem Lab Med 2007;45(6):700–7.

40. Stankovic AK. The laboratory is a key partner in assuring patient safety. Clin Lab Med 2004;24(4):1023–35.

41. Boone DJ. How can we make laboratory testing safer? Clin Chem Lab Med 2007; 45(6):708–11.

42. Golemboski K. Improving patient safety: lessons from other disciplines. Clin Lab Sci 2011;24(2):114–9.

43. Kay J. Technology to improve quality and accountability. Clin Chem Lab Med 2006;44(6):719–23.

44. Lippi G, Plebani M. Informatics aids to reduce failure rates in notification of abnormal outpatient test results. Arch Intern Med 2009;169(19):1815 [author reply: 1816–7].

45. Plebani M, Lippi G. Improving the post-analytical phase. Clin Chem Lab Med 2010;48(4):435–6.

46. Laposata ME, Laposata M, Van Cott EM, et al. Physician survey of a laboratory medicine interpretive service and evaluation of the influence of interpretations on laboratory test ordering. Arch Pathol Lab Med 2004;128(12):1424–7.

47. Plebani M. Interpretative commenting: a tool for improving the laboratory-clinical interface. Clin Chim Acta 2009;404(1):46–51.

48. Piva E, Plebani M. Interpretative reports and critical values. Clin Chim Acta 2009; 404(1):52–8.

Index

Note: Page numbers of article titles are in **boldface** type.

A

Absorbance measurement, 175
Absurdity checks, 155–156
Acceptable performance, 32–35
Accreditation, voluntary, 35–38
Accuracy, definition of, 127–128
Accuracy controls, **125–137**
    commutability and, 130–131
    definitions of, 126–128
    errors and, 128–129
    goals of, 125–126
    guidelines for use of, 133–134
    reagents for, 134–135
    reference materials for, 134–135
    traceability in, 129–130
    versus precision controls, 125–126, 130–133
Air contamination, detection of, 97
Albumin, patient population controls for, 143
Alternative quality control, 30
American College of American Pathologists, regulatory requirements of, 38
Analytical performance, **55–73**
    consistency across instruments in, 57
        evaluation of, 65–71
        limits of, 58–63
    detection limit in, 57
        evaluation of, 65–71
        limits of, 58–61
    linearity in, 57
        evaluation of, 64–70
        limits of, 55–59, 61
    precision in, 56–57
        evaluation of, 64, 66–70
        limits of, 57–60
    trueness in, 57
        evaluation of, 64, 66–70
        limits of, 58–61
Analytical quality management, 9–11
Analytical run, definition of, 16
Assayed controls, 132
Automatic quality control, 91

Clin Lab Med 33 (2013) 195–205
http://dx.doi.org/10.1016/S0272-2712(12)00149-7
0272-2712/13/$ – see front matter © 2013 Elsevier Inc. All rights reserved.

labmed.theclinics.com

W

Moving?

Make sure your subscription moves with you!

To notify us of your new address, find your **Clinics Account Number** (located on your mailing label above your name), and contact customer service at:

Email: journalscustomerservice-usa@elsevier.com

800-654-2452 (subscribers in the U.S. & Canada)
314-447-8871 (subscribers outside of the U.S. & Canada)

Fax number: 314-447-8029

Elsevier Health Sciences Division
Subscription Customer Service
3251 Riverport Lane
Maryland Heights, MO 63043

*To ensure uninterrupted delivery of your subscription, please notify us at least 4 weeks in advance of move.

Printed and bound by CPI Group (UK) Ltd, Croydon, CR0 4YY

03/10/2024

01040440-0002